REVERSING DIGESTION MISERY

Uncommon Cures for the Worst Gastrointestinal Problems!

Dr. David Williams

TABLE OF CONTENTS

Your Digestive Health Transformation Starts Here

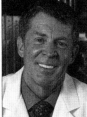

Dear Friend,

Your digestive system is your body's unsung hero. It breaks down the food you eat and sends critical nutrients into your bloodstream, sustaining all of your other organs and systems.

But, beyond this obvious role, your gastrointestinal (GI) tract is also a major player in your immune system. It's where your body sorts the good from the bad in what you've ingested, makes use of what's needed for your health and vitality, and eliminates the rest. It neutralizes pathogens with acids, enzymes, and friendly bacteria. And it ensures that other toxins move safely through your digestive organs and out of your body.

That's why, when something's amiss with your digestive system, your whole body suffers. Without healthy GI function, you open the door to nutritional deficiencies, increased absorption of toxins, poor immune function, inflammation, fatigue, and all manner of health conditions—from minor to life-threatening.

Unfortunately, digestive ailments and disorders have reached epidemic proportions in our country. It's estimated that 1 in 10 Americans suffer from heartburn at least once a week. More than 4 million Americans have frequent constipation, accounting for 2.5 million physician visits a year. 1 in 5 Americans has symptoms of irritable bowel syndrome (IBS), making it one of the most common disorders diagnosed by doctors. And, not counting skin cancers, colorectal cancer is the third most common cancer found in men and women in this country, with over 106,000 new cases diagnosed each year.

Digestive problems can have a profound effect on the quality of life. They bring on physical pain and misery coupled with emotional upset and embarrassment. It's a heavy burden to bear and people are shelling out *over 19 billion dollars* a year in prescription drugs and *over 5 billion dollars* in over-the-counter products trying to find relief.

According to a recent report from the US Department of Health and Human Services, 1 of every 10 Americans received at least one GI medication on an outpatient basis in 2007, compared with 1 of every 15 Americans in 1997. And this 60% increase went hand in hand with a whopping 170% increase in total expenditures on these medications.[1]

But most of these drugs only address the symptoms of digestive disorders, not the underlying causes. And for that simple reason, the problems (and drug company profits) will undoubtedly continue to grow.

Add to that the fact that many of these digestive health "solutions" have side effects that range from annoying to worrisome to life-threatening. And, ironically, a large number of the unwanted side effects are…additional digestive problems! So using these prescription and over-the-counter drugs can ultimately complicate your digestive distress rather than ease it.

Thankfully, your digestive health doesn't have to follow this dismal path. There are safe, natural, *proven* solutions that can help you rebuild a strong, capable digestive system. And most will do what years of over-the-counter or prescription medications never could—resolve your digestive complaints *and* boost your overall health.

In this book, I'll give you a brief overview of your amazing digestive system to help you better appreciate all it does for you. This short anatomy lesson will also enhance your understanding of how certain nutrients, techniques, or other solutions I recommend actually work to bring lasting relief from your digestive system ailments.

Next, I'll outline the four essential steps you need to take to nurture and fortify your digestive system, creating a solid foundation for digestive wellness. These are:

- Eating a healthy diet
- Drinking pure water
- Managing your stress and
- Creating balanced bacterial flora in your bowel

Then, I'll address six major digestive ailments that are plaguing our country's population, including:

- Acid Reflux/GERD
- Ulcers
- IBS—Irritable Bowel Syndrome
- Food Allergies
- IBD—Inflammatory Bowel Disease (including Crohn's and Ulcerative Colitis)
- Colorectal Cancer

For each, I'll give you details about the disorder and an action plan for addressing it, complete with dietary suggestions, nutrient recommendations, and techniques that have brought relief to others with this condition.

Many of these conditions share common symptoms—including heartburn, indigestion, nausea, excessive gas, diarrhea, and constipation. And in the next section of this book, I'll cover each of these symptoms, with my specific recommendations for ending the suffering that they bring.

If you're experiencing several of these digestive symptoms, but don't have a definitive diagnosis of a specific condition, then you'll want to skip directly to the Symptom section of the book so you can learn more about the symptoms you're experiencing and what to do about them immediately.

With these details in hand, you'll have what you've never had before…the tools to truly transform your digestive health so you can rediscover the joy of living in digestive comfort.

Yours in good health,

Dr. David Williams

P.S. To make it easy for you to implement my recommendations, I included a "Resources" section at the end of the book. There you'll find details on the specific brands and products I suggest, as well as where to go to find them.

PART I

The First Steps

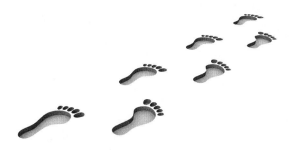

Getting to Know Your GI System

Your digestive system is a complex marvel of organs that work together physically and chemically to break down the food you ingest into nutrients it can absorb to nourish and energize your body's cells and systems, or excrete as waste outside the body.

The alimentary canal is the main part of the digestive system, where your food travels from start to finish and consists of your mouth, throat, esophagus, stomach, small intestine, large intestine, rectum, and anus. The average length of this GI tract in an adult male is 20–30 feet! Your digestive system also includes organs that lie outside this main pathway, including your pancreas, liver, and gallbladder.

Let's take a look at the journey that transpires within you at every meal.

Mouth and throat

When you take a bite of food, mucus membranes that line the mouth and ducts from your salivary glands in your cheeks, tongue, and under your jaw empty their contents into your mouth. Your saliva contains digestive enzymes that begin the process of breaking down the food you eat into its component parts.

Your teeth work to cut and grind your food into smaller, more easily digestible pieces, and your tongue not only tastes the food in your mouth, but serves to mix it up into a ball called a *bolus* and push it to the back of your mouth so you can swallow it.

Esophagus

Swallowing starts as a voluntary movement, but continues automatically with muscular contractions that create the wave-like motion that propels your food through the esophagus to your stomach. This movement is known as *peristalsis*, and occurs throughout your GI tract.

Your food's peristalsis-propelled trip through your 10–13 inch long esophagus takes less than 10 seconds. This thin-walled, muscular channel is lined with mucus membranes and has an upper esophageal sphincter (UES) at the top to keep food from going back into your throat, and a lower esophageal sphincter (LES), which opens to

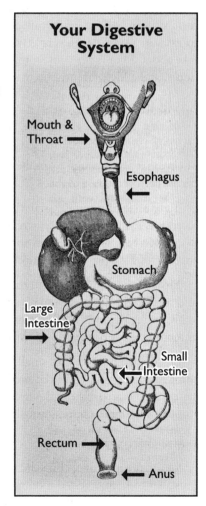

Your Digestive System

Mouth & Throat →

Esophagus ←

Stomach

Large Intestine →

Small Intestine

Rectum →

← Anus

release food into your stomach and then closes again to make sure caustic chemicals from your stomach don't make their way into the esophagus.

Stomach

Your stomach is a large, bean-shaped organ that receives food from the esophagus and then serves as a storage chamber of sorts. It uses rhythmic muscle contractions and digestive enzymes to continue breaking down the bolus into smaller nutrients that your body can use.

The cells lining the stomach secrete hydrochloric acid and the precursor of the enzyme pepsin. Both of these secretions help break down the proteins in your food into amino acids. Your stomach also secretes mucus to protect itself from these corrosive acids and enzymes.

Your stomach's high acidity doesn't just serve to break down food proteins, though. It also protects against infection by killing most bacteria that enter the stomach.

Food remains in your stomach for an average of 2–6 hours, in which time it's transformed into a sludgy liquid called *chyme*. The amount of time it takes for the stomach to work its magic depends largely on the type of food you eat. Healthy, whole foods take about 2 hours for your stomach to digest. A high-protein meal can take up to four hours, and a high-fat meal up to six hours.

Small intestine

Your stomach releases its chyme into the duodenum—the first segment of your small intestine—through the pyloric sphincter. This gatekeeper regulates the amount of chyme it lets through from the stomach each time, to keep the small intestine from becoming overwhelmed.

The duodenum pumps water into the mix to dilute the stomach acids and also receives enzymes from the pancreas, bile from the liver, and bile salts from the gallbladder, which help with digestion and absorption. In fact, absorption of nutrients is the small intestine's primary function.

Most of the duodenum and the remainder of the small intestine, is lined with folds and small projections called villi and microvilli, which increase the surface area to allow for greater nutrient absorption. It is in the small intestine where fats, starches, and proteins are broken down into absorbable acids, simple sugars, and amino acids.

Once broken down into small enough particles, useable nutrients can be absorbed through the thin lining of the small intestine into the bloodstream and lymphatic system to be carried throughout your body for fuel and functioning. The chyme's trip through the small intestine usually takes about 3–5 hours.

Large intestine

Your large intestine, also called the colon, is about four feet long and highly muscular to keep digested food moving along using peristalsis. The walls of the intestine also secrete mucus to facilitate this movement. Additionally, your large intestine reabsorbs up to 90% of the water and electrolytes remaining in the digested material, leaving behind solid fecal matter.

The time it takes for food to travel this last leg of its journey varies greatly, but is estimated to be between 4–72 hours.

Your colon is also home to vast colonies of bacteria. The "good" bacteria (or probiotics) help with digestion and absorption of nutrients, and also make important substances such as vitamin K. You will soon learn the far-reaching health benefits of maintaining proper amounts of these probiotics in your gut.

Meal Time!

How long does a meal take on its fantastic journey through your digestive system?

Transit Location	Transit Time
Esophagus	< 10 seconds
Stomach	2-6 hours
Small Intestine	3-5 hours
Large Intestine	4-72 hours
Total	9-83 hours

Rectum and anus

The final six inches of your colon make up your rectum. Fecal waste collects here until it reaches a point of fullness that signals the urge to defecate. The external anal sphincter is a muscle under voluntary control that sits at the bottom of your rectum. It keeps feces in place until you can reach a toilet.

When you're ready, you expel feces through your anus—the opening at the far end of your digestive tract. Your anus is formed partly from intestinal cells and partly from external skin.

? Did You Know...

Your GI tract is so efficient at breaking down and absorbing nutrients that your stools contain only a small amount of undigested food. Feces are largely made up of bacteria, bile, mucus, intestinal cells, and water.

Restoring Your Foundation for Digestive Health

In order to regain your digestive health, you must first lay a proper foundation to nurture and fortify your digestive system. This includes eating a healthy, balanced, easy-to-digest diet; drinking pure, clean water; managing your stress; and ensuring that you have balanced bacterial flora in your bowel.

Let's examine each of these digestive health foundation "building blocks" in more detail.

Eat a healthy, balanced, easy-to-digest diet

The quality and balance of the foods you eat have a profound effect on every system in your body, but none more than your digestive system. This just makes good, plain sense, since your digestive system is responsible for breaking down these foods, extracting the nutrients your body needs to stay healthy and vital, and efficiently eliminating the rest.

If you don't put quality, nutritious foods into your system, you won't get the vitamins, minerals, and other critical nutrients you need to protect and promote your good health—including that of your digestive system. Furthermore, eating a diet high in sugar, refined carbohydrates, and fat, but low in fiber and whole foods will prevent your digestive system from operating optimally, throw off the delicate balance of bacteria in your intestines, and exacerbate your digestive woes.

For instance, we now consume less fiber and more refined carbohydrates than at any other time in history. Both of these habits slow digestive transit time, allowing toxins to sit in your body far too long and providing fuel for harmful bacteria strains.

Reshaping your dietary and eating habits isn't necessarily complicated, but does require commitment. After all, old habits can be hard to break. But, the payoff is well worth the effort—not only in the new digestive comfort you'll enjoy, but also the increase in physical and mental energy you'll experience.

The basics of a healthy, digestive system–supporting diet boil down to this: <u>Focus on nutritious, low-fat, high-fiber foods, with an emphasis on fresh vegetables and fruits, lean proteins, and whole grains</u>. In addition, there are a few dietary "secrets" that I want to share because they're especially important for healthy, comfortable digestion.

Here are the details to help you create a diet that's good for your digestive health and overall wellness…

Give dietary priority to wholesome plant foods

Plant foods are low in fat, moderate in protein, and contain an abundance of vitamins, minerals, essential fatty acids, and protective phytochemicals. Simply eating

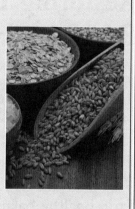

more healthy fruits, vegetables, seeds, and grains can dramatically change your body's nutrient levels, which benefits your digestive system and all other systems in your body.

Plants are also nature's only source of dietary fiber. Insoluble fiber, found in whole grains and the skins and outer coatings of seeds, fruits, and legumes, promotes bowel regularity, which is critical for the efficient removal of toxins from your body. For this reason, getting sufficient insoluble fiber is important to your digestive health and immune health.

Fruits, vegetables, seeds, and grains also contain soluble fiber, which not only nourishes and strengthens your colon so it can perform at its best, but also lowers cholesterol and helps maintain healthy blood sugar levels.

Look for low-fat, high-quality lean protein

The protein in your digestive health–supporting diet should come from lean sources like poultry, fish, egg whites, nonfat yogurt, beans, and grains. Several times a week, try to eat wild-caught coldwater fish, such as salmon, mackerel, herring, and cod, which are rich in healthy omega-3 fatty acids in addition to being good sources of protein. And avoid the saturated fat in red meat.

Make sure you're getting sufficient omega-3 fatty acids

The diet of our ancestors offered a good balance of fats and oils from both plants and animals—including the proper ratio of omega-3 and omega-6 essential fatty acids. These fatty acids are your body's raw material for other fatty acids and compounds essential for controlling a wide variety of bodily functions—including healthy digestion. In fact, a common problem stemming from out-of-balance fatty acids is food allergies.

Omega-6 and omega-3 fatty acids are not neutral, so for good health they must be eaten in a relatively fixed ratio. The ratio of omega-6 fatty acids to omega-3 fatty

Chia—An Excellent Source of Fiber and Omega-3 Fatty Acids

I can vividly remember watching late-night commercials in the 1980s and hearing "Ch-ch-ch-chia!" as sprouts were shown growing out of a funky terra cotta Chia Pet. At the time, the last thing that would have crossed my mind was eating chia seeds as a food. Little did I know.

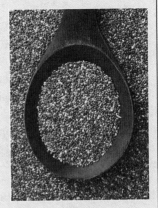

Chia (*Salvia hispanica*) was first cultivated in the southern part of Mexico next to Guatemala. It has a long history of use among the Aztec and Mayan cultures, and is now gaining recognition as a modern-day miracle food.

Oil from chia has the highest proportion of omega-3 fatty acids of any plant known. It's naturally pest-free, so it doesn't require the use of pesticides or herbicides for growing. And it contains a naturally high level of antioxidants—including caffeic acid, chlorogenic acid, and quercetin—that protect it from rancidity.

When it comes to omega-3 content, chia gives you a lot of "bang for your buck":

Omega-3 Content per 100 Grams

Food	Omega-3 content
Salmon, wild Pacific	1.7 grams
Sardines	1.6 grams
Flax	22.8 grams
Chia	24.3 grams

In addition to having a high omega-3 content, chia is a good source of protein and calcium, low in sodium, lower in net carbohydrates than other grains, and an excellent source of both soluble and insoluble fiber.

The easiest way to use it is to simply sprinkle it in salads, over vegetables, or on top of other foods. I suggest 2 tablespoons a day for adults and 1 tablespoon for children.

Chia sources I recommend are Ruth's Hemp Foods (*ruthshempfoods.com* or 877-359-4508) and Natural Remi-Teas (*naturalremi-teas.com* or 1-866-428-0575).

acids in our ancestors' diet was typically a healthy four to one (4:1). Today that ratio is anywhere from 20:1 to 25:1.

This imbalance is due, in part, to the popularity of vegetable oils in our diet, which have abundant omega-6 fatty acids. Another drastic change has been in our country's farming practices. Our ancestors ate livestock that grazed mainly on grass and other plant foods. The meat from such animals is leaner and has up to five times the omega-3 content of meat from feedlot- and cage-raised animals that are typical of today's livestock.

Likewise, many of the most popular dietary fish, such as salmon, trout, catfish, shrimp, and others, are now being farmed instead of fresh caught, which dramatically lowers their omega-3 essential fatty acid content. Instead of getting their normal diet of omega-3–rich components such as minnows, krill, algae, or insects, these fish are being fed omega-6–rich grains and grain byproducts.

To boost your omega-3 fatty acid intake, make sure the meat and poultry you choose is from farms with free-range feeding practices and that the fish you eat is wild-caught, not farmed.

Even more important, try to eat more dark green leafy vegetables. Other good sources of healthy omega-3 fatty acids are seed oils from flax, hemp, pumpkin, and black currant. And a surprising "newcomer" to the omega-3 scene is a food of high standing from centuries past—chia. (See previous page for more details on this.)

Stay away from processed sugar

It's also important that you stay away from processed sugar. Aside from being difficult to digest, it contributes to weight gain and wreaks havoc with your immune system by depleting your adrenal glands. Sugar has also been shown to slow down the mobility of white blood cells and reduce the production of certain disease-fighting hormones.[2]

Sugar hides in nearly all processed foods, particularly in the form of high fructose corn syrup. To avoid it, try to stick with fresh foods as much as possible and make sure you read labels carefully on the packaged food items you do put in your grocery cart.

If you have a sweet tooth, bypass the processed sugar and satisfy it with one of these two healthy, natural sweeteners:

Stevia

This natural sweetener comes from a plant found in Paraguay and Brazil, and has been safely used in South America for centuries, as well as throughout Japan and the Pacific Rim. Several attributes set Stevia apart from other sweeteners. First, it retards the growth of dental plaque. Second, it doesn't support the growth of *Candida* (the yeast that's behind most yeast infections). And third, it has the unique ability of helping to regulate blood sugar levels. This makes Stevia one of the few sweeteners that can be used safely by people with diabetes. You'll find Stevia sold under the brand name "Truvia," and it is widely available online and in health food stores.

Xylitol

This sugar replacement, which was discovered in the 1800s, has been found to help prevent tooth decay and even reduce the incidence of ear infections in children. Research suggests that this is because *Streptococcus mutans (S. mutans)*, which is a common type of bacteria that resides in dental plaque and the mucus membranes lining the mouth, nose, and throat, can't properly digest xylitol. Xylitol impairs the bacteria's ability to adhere to surfaces, makes it less virulent, and also decreases its numbers.

Xylitol powder can be used as a direct substitute for sugar in all types of cooking and baking. It measures like sugar, and it's practically as sweet as sugar. It's available through numerous online retailers and in many health food stores.

Fabulous fermented food

Lactic acid–fermented foods were dietary staples for thousands of years, and lactic acid–fermented cabbage has been revered as one of the most beneficial healing agents throughout recorded history.

Decades before antibiotics, cabbage juice was successfully used to prevent or heal peptic ulcers. In one recent study, cabbage juice alone had a cure rate of over 92 percent in the treatment of these ulcers, compared to about 32 percent with a placebo or other treatment. The dosage in the study consisted of only 50 cc of raw cabbage juice from a quart of freshly pressed cabbage.[3]

Unfortunately, in the last 100 years, most of the more beneficial fermented foods have fallen from favor. Much of the problem has to do with the way we now preserve foods, particularly vegetables.

When fresh vegetables weren't as readily available throughout the year, they were often preserved through fermentation. Nowadays, thanks to improved transportation and storage techniques, we can buy various vegetables all year around. And when it comes to preserving vegetables, freezing and canning have become the methods of choice.

While these techniques help retain vitamin content and provide a high degree of convenience, they do little to provide important digestive health benefits.

Proper bacterial flora in your gut

Lactic acid–fermented foods help to maintain and nurture the proper bacterial flora in your lower bowel. And mounting research has shown beyond a shadow of a doubt that this is one of the most important factors in maintaining your good health.

In fact, creating a healthy bacterial balance in your gut is one of the four building blocks for a strong digestive health foundation, and I'll give you more details on this further along in this book.

But, a brief summary is that probiotics—the "good" bacteria—work to crowd out harmful bacteria and promote healthy digestion by improving nutrient absorption and encouraging regular bowel movements. They also support the immune system by helping to block pathogens and other toxins from being reabsorbed into your body and by minimizing the toxic byproducts of the bad bacteria in your bowels.

Balanced stomach acids

Lactic acid–fermented foods also help balance the production of acid in the stomach. When the stomach produces less hydrochloric acid, fermented foods help increase acidity of gastric juices. When there is an overproduction of acid, they protect the stomach and intestinal lining.

As we get older, our production of the digestive juices and enzymes required for proper digestion begin to decrease, making stomach upset more frequent. Fermented foods can help make up for this loss and relieve indigestion.

Improved acetylcholine production

Finally, lactic acid–fermented foods produce acetylcholine, a neurotransmitter that increases bowel motility and promotes the release of digestive juices and enzymes from the stomach, pancreas, and gallbladder—all which are necessary for optimal digestive function.

? Did You Know…

In addition to benefits it provides to your gastrointestinal system, acetylcholine has also been linked to the phase of sleep called rapid eye movement (REM). REM occurs when you experience the deepest and most beneficial sleep.

Since lactic acid-fermented foods produce acetylcholine, it stands to reason that eating these foods regularly might also enhance your sleep habits, which can dramatically improve your overall health.

Even though fermented foods are no longer a common dietary staple, I can't over-stress the need for you to get them into your daily diet. One of the easiest and best ways to do that is with sauerkraut.

Sauerkraut

Making and eating your own sauerkraut with lactic acid–fermented cabbage is an easy, fun, and inexpensive process that I encourage everyone to do, especially if you have digestive concerns.

Keep in mind that, due to their acidity, lactic acid–fermented vegetables should be used as a complement to meals and not eaten in large quantities. Consistency is the key, so eat small amounts—3 to 4 tablespoons—on a daily basis.

There are several books currently in print on the subject of lactic acid–fermentation as a method of preserving food, but my favorite is *Nourishing Traditions* by Sally Fallon. (It's available from *Amazon.com*, Barnes & Noble or New Trends Publishing at 1-877-707-1776.)

The book has a wealth of information on various health topics and the chapter on lactic acid-fermented foods contains savory recipes for sauerkraut, pickled cucumbers, garlic, beets, radish, corn relish, potatoes, various chutneys, Korean kimchi, and more.

Yogurt—your other easy probiotic source

Eating fermented foods is an easy way to get all-important probiotics into your system, as is eating live-culture yogurt.

Unfortunately, most of the yogurt products available here in America are laden with too much sugar and artificial ingredients. Plus, even if a yogurt package says the product contains "live and active cultures," the probiotic benefits are often lost during manufacturing, delivery, and storage of the yogurts on your grocer's shelves.

A far better (and more delicious) solution is homemade yogurt. I've experimented with doing this from scratch and it can be tricky business, so I recommend using a yogurt maker instead.

An Easy Way to Make Your Own Sauerkraut

Dr. Williams' Favorite Recipe

(Makes 1 quart)

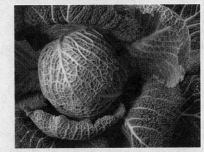

- 4 cups shredded cabbage, loosely packed
- 1 tsp. juniper berries
- ½ tsp. cumin seeds
- ½ tsp. mustard seeds
- 2 tsp. sea salt
- 2 Tbsp. liquid whey* (if not available, add an additional 1 teaspoon salt)
- 1 cup filtered water (Don't use chlorinated tap water. Chlorine can destroy lactic microbial organisms and prevent fermentation.)

In a bowl, mix cabbage, juniper berries, cumin, and mustard seeds. Mash or pound with a wooden mallet for several minutes to release juices. Place in a quart-sized wide-mouth Mason jar and pack down. Mix water with salt and whey and pour into jar. Add more water, if needed, to cover cabbage. There should be about one inch of space between the top of the cabbage and the top of the jar.

Place a lid on the jar and close tightly. Lacto-fermentation is an anaerobic (without oxygen) process and the presence of oxygen, once fermentation has begun, will ruin the final product. Keep at room temperature for three days. Transfer to a root cellar or the top shelf of your refrigerator. The sauerkraut can be eaten immediately, but it improves with age.

Note: It's normal for white spots or a white film to form on the surface of the liquid covering the sauerkraut. This is a form of yeast called kahm. Although it's totally harmless, it can impart a bad taste to the cabbage. I would recommend removing it gently with a spoon before eating the sauerkraut.

* If you use whey, it must be in the liquid form, not powdered. You can make your own whey by pouring yogurt into cheesecloth, a coffee filter, or a clean kitchen towel. Capture the whey liquid as it drips into another container. Using whey allows you to decrease the amount of salt needed and improves consistency. It is naturally rich in both lactic acid and lactic acid–producing bacteria.

There are many brands on the market today, and I've tried quite a few, but I believe the best of the bunch is the Euro-Cuisine Yogurt Maker, which can be purchased from a variety of online retailers. It's extremely easy to use and lets me make a batch of delicious, healthy yogurt that lasts throughout the week.

If you don't want to make your own yogurt, there are two store-bought brands that I recommend and which are likely to contain beneficial bacteria that are still alive and kicking. These are Stoneyfield Farm Organic Yogurt (widely available in grocery stores and health food stores) and White Mountain Bulgarian Yogurt, which is sold mostly throughout the Midwest and East Coast regions.

Homemade health from bone broth

In addition to fermented food, another important dietary component has regrettably become an endangered species—the amino acid glycine. This is unfortunate because glycine is a component of many body functions and a deficiency can result in a wide variety of health problems, including digestive ailments.

Gelatin, the protein substance made from boiling animal bones, skins, and tendons, is one of the richer natural sources of glycine. And I believe the glycine shortage in our diets is a direct result of the decreased popularity of making and consuming bone broths.

I've seen people with all types of digestive and food allergy problems get lasting relief with the simple addition of bone broth to their diets. And bone broths are easy to make.

Simple Steps for a Healthful Soup

To make your own bone broth, begin by placing the bones from organically raised fish, poultry, beef, lamb, or pork into a large stainless steel or porcelain pot. (I don't recommend aluminum because it can leach into the broth.) The bones can be raw or cooked, and they can be stripped of meat or still contain meat remnants and skin.

Cover the bones with water. Add a couple of tablespoons of <u>one</u> of the following per quart of water: apple cider vinegar, red or white wine vinegar, or lemon juice. Gently stir and then let it sit for about 30 minutes to let the acid go to work.

Then bring the water to a boil and immediately cut back to a slow, steady simmer. Cover and continue to simmer for 4 to 6 hours for fish, 6 to 8 hours for poultry, and 12 to 18 hours for the other types of bones.

Keep a lid on the pot to avoid having to add water (but add water if and when necessary). If you want to add vegetables, strain the liquid first and then add the vegetables for about the last 30 minutes of simmering. Feel free to add other items—such as salt, pepper, butter, or olive oil—to enhance the flavor.

A slow cooker works well for bone broth since the temperature is generally low enough that the lid will keep in the steam and it won't require much attention. However, I've found that slow cookers generally take about ⅓ longer than when I cook on the stove.

If you want just the broth, strain the liquid through a colander and consume it immediately either by sipping as a tea or soup, or making it into gravy. You can also use it as the liquid to cook rice, beans, or grains.

The broth can be stored in the refrigerator for about five days, or stored frozen for several months. (I generally pour the cooled liquid into quart freezer bags and freeze those. When I want some broth, I simply open the bag and reheat the broth in a pot.)

Note: *Never cook or reheat the broth (or gelatin) in the microwave. Certain amino acids may convert into forms that can be toxic to the body when microwaved.*

Change the way you buy and eat your food, too

To get the biggest benefits from the foods you eat, try to buy organic whenever you can. Certainly it costs a bit more and sometimes spoils more quickly, but your health is definitely worth the investment.

One of the biggest concerns I have about many foods, especially most of the fruits and vegetables available these days, is their exposure to pesticides and other environmental toxins. Eating organic will help you avoid these and keep your digestive and immune systems from having to process them.

The US Department of Agriculture recently tested more than 27,000 food samples and found pesticide residue (primarily methyl parathion) in a number of other popular fresh fruits and veggies. The most contaminated were domestic and imported peaches, grapes, apples, pears, spinach, green beans, and fresh and frozen winter squash. Most of the pesticides were concentrated on or just below the skin. So, when buying these particular items, I'd definitely recommend going the organic route.

Other research, reported in the *Journal of Alternative and Complementary Medicine*, noted that organic crops contained significantly more vitamin C, iron, magnesium, and phosphorus, and significantly less nitrates, than conventional crops. The study found a 372 percent increase in selenium content in the organic crops over the conventional ones. It also showed that organics contained a better quality and higher content of other nutritionally significant materials, with lower amounts of some heavy metals.

If you don't have organic options for these fruits and vegetables, either peel them or wash them in mild, soapy water or a produce rinse to thoroughly remove the residue. (In fact, I recommend doing this to all your fruits and vegetables. It can eliminate dirt and germs as well as chemicals.)

In addition to improving the quality and kinds of food you eat, try to change the *way* you eat, too. Consume 5 or 6 smaller meals a day rather than 2 or 3 large ones. Don't eat more, just spread it out. This will promote healthier digestion as well as help keep your blood sugar levels constant throughout the day, keep your energy levels up, and curb your cravings for sugary "pick-me-up" foods.

Eat your largest meal in the morning and your lightest meal in the early evening. And be especially aware of what is considered a portion of food.

A few examples of serving sizes are:

- Vegetables or fruit—the size of your fist
- Beans, pasta, rice, or pretzels—one rounded handful
- Cheese—size of 4 stacked dice
- Fish—the size of your checkbook
- Meat—the size of your palm (not counting your fingers)

Juice It!

One of the simplest ways to get the nutrients your body needs to thrive is to incorporate fresh juice into your diet. Juices provide a ready supply of vital vitamins, minerals, and other healing compounds to nourish your body and boost your immunity. And it eases the work load of your digestive system.

Grinding up vegetables or fruits to make juice breaks down the cellulose of the plant, releasing nutrients and quickly making them available to your body's cells. What's more, because juice takes little energy to digest, almost all of its nutrients and energy stores remain to be used by your body. For example, you'd have to eat eight carrots to get the same vitamin content found in a mere six ounces of carrot juice.

Most bottled juice is a nutrition nightmare, containing artificial colors and added sugar. Unless it's squeezed in the store where it's sold, store-bought juice must be pasteurized, a process that destroys enzymes and some nutrients.

Making your own juice at home guarantees freshness. But, once a fruit or vegetable goes through a juicer, natural enzymes in the food begin to break down the nutrients, so be sure to drink the juice within 30 minutes of preparation to get its maximum health benefits.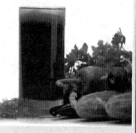

There are numerous juicers on the market that make the job of juicing easy and the clean-up afterward simple. The one I use at home is the L'Equip and is widely available at department stores and through online retailers.

Drink pure, clean water

A second building block for creating a health digestive health foundation is keeping your body hydrated. This is such a basic step for good health that's it's often overlooked, which is a big mistake. Aside from air, water is probably the only thing you ingest each and every day of your life.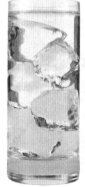

It's essential for your existence. In fact, roughly 57 percent of your total body weight is water and every bodily system—including your digestive system—depends on the movement of water through your cells, tissues, and organs.

Experts agree that you should get a minimum of eight 8-ounce glasses of pure, clean water each day.

Be wary of your water sources

The real trick here might not be training yourself to consume this amount of water each day, but finding a source of water that's truly clean and pure.

Even "approved" drinking water, under the Environmental Protection Agency (EPA) standards, may contain specified amounts of lead, arsenic, mercury, radioactive particles, and a long list of other poisons that come into direct contact with your digestive system organs and can also accumulate in your body tissue, both of which can eventually lead to serious illness.

Although millions have turned to bottled water for its advertised purity and convenience, it isn't much better than tap water. One FDA survey found that 31 percent of 52 brands tested were tainted with bacteria, 29 percent of bottling facilities visited exhibited poor manufacturing practices, and 31 percent had significant "deviations" in their water testing.

Even worse, the bottles themselves may be contributing to the contamination of the water inside. Bisphenol A (BPA) is a component of the plastic used to make many water bottles. Researchers discovered that BPA can leach out of plastic bottles into the liquid they contain and, once inside your body, it mimics estrogen and can wreak all sorts of havoc in your body's endocrine system.

?

Did You Know...

Thirty-five percent of the reported gastrointestinal illnesses among tap water drinkers were water related and preventable.

—Centers for Disease Control and Prevention

Distillation is a superior solution for pure, clean water

Since you can't rely on bottled water, municipal water treatment facilities, the government, or anyone else to provide you with safe water, the only solution is to take advantage of water filtration technology for your own home.

My first choice for safe drinking water is distillation because it safely removes all contaminants, leaving behind pure H_2O just as Mother Nature intended. There are critics of distillation, but I think it is the very best way to go when it comes to all-around water purification.

Distillation is a fairly simple process. Water is heated until it boils and turns to steam. The boiling action kills the various bacteria and other pathogens, and as the steam rises it leaves behind waste material, minerals, heavy metals, and other heavier contaminants. The water vapor is then cooled and returns to its liquid form.

A good distillation system will remove every kind of bacteria, virus, parasite, and pathogen, as well as pesticides, herbicides, organic and inorganic chemicals, heavy metals (dissolved or otherwise), and even radioactive contaminants. It's the *only* purification method I know of that removes *all* of these impurities. The water distiller that I prefer and have used for years myself is the Waterwise 9000 (Visit *waterwise.com* or call 1-800-874-9028 to order.)

Stress relief

A third building block for a strong digestive health foundation is stress relief. Some people find this surprising but, without a doubt, your digestive system is intricately connected to your emotions.

Just think about a time when you felt nervous, afraid, angry, or overwhelmed. Chances are one of the places in your body that took the brunt of those strong feelings was your gut.

Butterflies in the stomach or a stomach tied in knots are common ways to describe the way you feel in stressful situations. It's no surprise that they call emotionally charged moments "gut-wrenching." And extreme stress can bring on real digestive symptoms, like diarrhea, stomach cramps, even vomiting.

Second only to your brain in number of nerves

One of the reasons why stressful emotions can lead to digestive issues is that your GI tract is rich in nerves and highly influenced by them. Your gut is controlled by the enteric nervous system, which consists of approximately 100 million nerves—the largest area of nerves outside the brain. For this reason, the gut is sometimes called "the little brain."

Your enteric nervous system operates much like your central nervous system, communicating with neurons and chemical neurotransmitters. And the two systems use common pathways along your sympathetic and parasympathetic nervous systems.

An age-old response to modern day stressors spells digestive upset

Another reason your GI tract can take a beating in the face of stress is that your body is still programmed to react to stress in a primitive way.

When you encounter a stressful situation, your body is flooded with "fight or flight" hormones, like cortisol and epinephrine, which—among other things—reduces gastrointestinal secretions and redirects blood flow from your digestive tract to your head, heart, and lungs in order to prepare your body to take action.

This reflexive response served a person well in the age-old time when stress usually came from a predator, like a bear in the woods, and fight or flight was an appropriate response. In today's world, however, your stress is more likely to come from work deadlines, family commitments, money issues, or relationship strains than from a bear, but the chemicals that flood your body are the same.

This chemical assault—especially if it continues day after day—can compromise your physical, mental, and emotional well-being. As you know, it can lead to digestive distress, but it can also contribute to insomnia, anxiety, depression, headaches, and muscle pain. If left unchecked, it can even lead to heart disease, hypertension, immune system problems, and reproductive disorders.

A vicious cycle

While stress can cause digestive system problems, the reverse is also true. Chronic or even occasional symptoms such as gas, bloating, cramping, diarrhea, constipation, or worse, can not only cause physical discomfort, but also emotional pain. These conditions can be embarrassing, isolating, worrisome, and stressful.

It's a vicious cycle and your health is the victim.

Find your own best way to manage stress

Clearly, it's vitally important to find a way to handle your stress so it doesn't negatively impact your digestive system or overall well-being. But managing stress is a highly individual process. What works for one person may have no place in another's life.

So, take some time to consider what stress-reducing steps might work for your personality and life circumstances. Here are some proven techniques that have helped others relieve stress and find an inner calm.

Deep breathing

Because breathing is automatic, you probably don't put much thought into it. But for relaxation, there's a special breathing technique you should employ. It's called abdominal breathing or deep breathing, and it's more effective at bringing oxygen to all tissues of your body.

Deep breathing helps relax your entire body, strengthens the muscles in your chest and abdomen, helps you burn calories more efficiently, and leaves you feeling calm, yet energized.

Whenever you feel tense, take a 3–5 minute break for deep breathing. Here's how:

1. Lie flat on your back with your knees pulled up. Keep your feet slightly apart.

2. Inhale deeply through your nose. As you breathe in, allow your stomach to relax so the air flows into your abdomen. Your stomach should balloon out as you breathe in.

3. Visualize your lungs filling up with energy so your chest swells out.

4. Exhale deeply.

5. As you breathe out, let your stomach and chest fall in. Imagine air coming out from your abdomen and then from your lungs.

Exercise

Abundant research has shown that exercise releases tension in your body and can release emotional tension as well.

Also, by improving your health, well-being, and self-image, exercise bolsters your body's ability to handle stress. And, depending on the type of exercise you choose, it can bring social benefits (like being part of a sports team) or meditative benefits (like you can achieve with yoga and T'ai Chi).

Laughter

Scientific studies have shown that children laugh about 400 times a day while adults laugh only about 15 times a day. That's a shame for the adults, since studies find that laughter lowers levels of cortisol and helps regulate heart rate and blood pressure.

Even the mere act of smiling has its benefits. Smiling sends a message to your brain to release endorphins, which are substances that relieve pain and give a sense of pleasure, peace, and well-being.

Try adding laughter to your life with funny movies and books. Go to a comedy club or make a point to spend time with friends and loved ones who make you smile.

Prayer and spirituality

Countless people over the centuries have turned to prayer for a sense of reassurance and calm. And a growing body of evidence points to the beneficial health effects of prayer and spirituality. This doesn't mean you have to be religious. You can find spirituality in a quiet walk in the woods or during the peaceful moments before you drift off to sleep.

Meditation

As meditation has become better known in Western cultures, scientists have begun to quantify its physical benefits in hundreds of studies. In one study of health insurance statistics, meditators had 87 percent fewer hospitalizations for heart disease, 55 percent fewer for benign and malignant tumors, and 30 percent fewer for infectious diseases. The meditators had more than 50 percent fewer doctor visits than did non-meditators.[4]

To start your meditation practice, find a quiet place and turn off your cell phone and other distractions. Don't allow yourself to be disturbed for at least 20 minutes. Next, pick a focus word or brief phrase that's meaningful to you. Some examples are "one," "peace," "shalom" or "om."

Then, sit comfortably, close your eyes, relax your body and mind, and breathe in through your nose and out through your mouth. As you are breathing out, say your word silently to yourself. Don't worry about thoughts coming in and out of your mind. Gently release them and return to the repetition. To achieve relaxation, use this technique for at least 10 to 15 minutes a day.

Music

Dr. Frederick Tims, chair of the music therapy program at Michigan State University, reports that clinical observations show that music produces more alpha rhythms in the brain. These particular rhythms are associated with relaxation.

Music is also believed to produce more endorphins, the body's natural painkillers. In addition to all of this, music shows potential for bolstering the immune system by regulating natural body rhythms and lowering levels of corticosteroids, including cortisol. So, choose the type of music you enjoy most and listen up.

Holistic health practices

Consider modalities such as chiropractic adjustments, acupuncture, or acupressure to help ease stress and improve wellness. These have long histories of success for a variety of health conditions.

Create balanced bacterial flora in your bowel

In my discussion about creating a healthy diet, I touched on the importance of nurturing healthy bacteria in your gut, and recommended that you eat fermented foods and live-culture yogurt on a regular basis to help with this.

Less Stress with More ZZZZ's

Getting sufficient sleep isn't just a nicety—it's critical to your overall good health. That's because sleep is the critical period when your body rests and rejuvenates. And when you don't get enough sleep, it affects your stress levels.

According to sleep researchers, there are 5 different stages of sleep that a person should recycle through every one to two hours nightly. Two of these stages are directly involved in the physiological immune system, and one is essential for emotional health, which impacts stress levels that, in turn, affect the immune system.[5]

Unfortunately, the struggle to get a good night's sleep is an exhausting battle shared by many. In fact, a random survey conducted by The National Sleep Foundation found that 76% of all Americans have trouble falling alseep.[6]

Others can get to sleep, but find themselves waking in the wee hours of the morning and not being able to fall back asleep. This same poll found that the number of people who say they're getting eight hours of sleep on a regular basis has decreased, from 38 percent in 2001 to 28 percent today.

To help ease your stress and aid your digestive function, follow these "good sleep tips" provided by the National Sleep Foundation:

- Maintain a standard, relaxing bedtime routine
- Stick to regular sleep times
- Keep bedrooms dark, cool, and quiet
- Make sure pillows, mattresses, and bedding are comfortable
- Exercise regularly, but stop at least three hours before bedtime
- Avoid caffeinated beverages (and for adults, alcohol) at least eight hours before turning in
- Keep work, computers, and televisions out of bedrooms

I also suggest that you:

- Avoid less obvious sources of caffeine, like chocolate, chocolate-flavored foods, soft drinks, and salt, which can act as a mild stimulant to the adrenal glands.
- Take a look at the medications you're using. One of the biggest detriments to sleep is the widespread use of both over-the-counter and prescription drugs. Even seemingly harmless sinus and nasal congestion medications can be strong nervous system stimulants that can interfere with sleep.
- Never accept a new prescription from your doctor until you've given him or her a complete list of drugs that you're taking, including over-the-counter medications. Anytime you develop a new symptom after starting a new drug, consider the new drug as the culprit until you prove otherwise.

But, even taking these steps may not be enough. There are dozens of reasons why, but let me give you a few of the biggest: Stress. Hidden toxins in your food. Chemicals and pathogens in your water. And the overuse of antibiotics.

All of these kill the "friendly" bacteria in your gut by the *billions*. And, because your body can't manufacture friendly bacteria on its own, you have to replace them from an outside source. That's why I strongly encourage you to take a daily probiotic supplement.

But, before I give you the details on exactly what you should look for in a quality probiotic supplement, let me cover a few more facts on the super-sized job these tiny bacteria do for your digestive and overall good health.

Tiny but mighty

Your digestive system—primarily your small and large intestines—are teeming with over 100 trillion bacteria. Experts have estimated that if you lined these bacteria up, they would stretch twice around the equator. That's almost 50,000 miles.

As you now know, there are the bacterial "bad guys" that can cause digestive upset and worse, and there are the probiotic "good guys" that are absolutely essential for your health and survival. These probiotics help digest the food you eat and break down dairy products for easier digestion. They work to prevent constipation and diarrhea. They even help to fight viruses.

Research has shown that the bacteria lining your intestines help to form a barrier that prevents pathogens from entering your body. This is particularly important in your large intestines, where fecal matter accumulates before being expelled from your body. Without a strong bacterial barrier in place, toxins from your feces can be reabsorbed into your body, adding to the already significant demands placed on your immune system each day.

Preventing the mayhem of toxic metabolites

Perhaps even more worrisome than fecal toxins are the toxic metabolites that bad bacteria can create. Pathogenic bacteria can enter your digestive system through your nose and mouth, and if they survive the trip through the acids and enzymes of the upper GI tract, they'll find a perfect home in your colon. It's a warm, moist, nutrient-rich environment that lacks oxygen and strong digestive fluids, making it an ideal place for bacteria to grow and flourish.

Without balanced bacteria in your colon, these pathogenic bacteria can gain a true foothold and will then constantly spew their toxic metabolites into your body. This places your immune system in a constant battle just to keep things under control. Proper flora in your bowels will prevent this unhealthy situation from becoming a reality in your body.

A health enhancer as well as protector

It's quite clear how probiotics work to protect your intestinal health and immune system function. But, they also serve as health enhancers, not just protectors.

Specifically, a healthy bacterial lining in your intestines actually improves the digestion of foods and the absorption of essential nutrients that feed and nourish every cell, organ, and system in your body. They even work to boost your body's natural vitamin production.

Add "Pre's" for Your "Pro's"

Prebiotics are non-digestible foods that help probiotics to grow and proliferate. The most common form of prebiotics is soluble fiber, and it's sometimes referred to as "fermentable fiber." This fiber makes its way through your digestive system relatively intact and, when it reaches your intestines, it helps create an environment where good bacteria can flourish.

Excellent food sources of prebiotics are: artichokes, bananas, barley, berries, chicory, flax, garlic, greens (including dandelion, chard and kale), honey, leeks, legumes, onions, and whole grains—especially oatmeal.

What to look for in a quality probiotic

Now that the word is out about probiotics and how important they are for proper digestion, immune system health, and overall wellness, many nutritional supplement manufacturers are jumping on the bandwagon and flooding the market with probiotic products that may very well be worthless. Certainly, you don't want to waste your time and money, or go another day with digestive discomfort, by taking a product that just doesn't live up to its promises.

That's why you should make sure the probiotic you choose has these important features:

- **Formulated with "pearl" or "beadlet" technology, or in a controlled-release tablet** to ensure that at least a billion of the live bacteria survive your stomach acids and arrive in your gut ready to take action.

- **Includes at least these three top probiotic strains:**

  L. acidophilus—the most important "good guy" for the small intestine. Helps maintain healthy intestinal walls and promote proper nutrient absorption. Also aids with dairy digestion.

  B. longum—acts as a cellular "SWAT" team by patrolling your large intestine and destroying bad bacteria as well as blocking toxins from being reabsorbed into your body. Also helps break down carbohydrates, aids in proper nutrient absorption, and supports your immune health.

  B. bifidum—the "Dairy King." This important bacterium works in both your small and large intestines and is critical for the healthy digestion of dairy products, which is especially important as you grow older and your natural ability to digest dairy declines.

- **Has a stated expiration date.** Expiration dates on nutritional supplements are strictly voluntary. But, if you don't see one, you should question its quality. With an expressed expiration date, the supplement manufacturer is letting you know that the ingredients should be active and potent until that time.

- **Comes with a money-back guarantee.** Always insist on this for any supplement you take, including your probiotic. If the probiotic you choose delivers the one billion or more healthy, live bacteria to your intestines as promised, then you should feel a dramatic difference in your digestive health and overall wellness. If you don't, send it back for a refund and find another product that does deliver.

I recommend an Enzy product called Pearls IC that contains 1 billion CFU among six different bacteria. There is also a Jarrow product called Jarrow-Dophilus EPS which contains 5 billion CFU among eight bacteria. Both are widely available in health food stores, or from *iHerb.com* (no phone ordering for iHerb).

❖ ❖ ❖

Support Our Troops...with Bacteria!

Recently, I ran across a study showing that infectious gastrointestinal disorders are among the biggest risks to our military troops who are deployed overseas. Every month, about 30 percent get infectious diarrhea. Those who had experienced even just one incident had six times the risk for subsequent functional diarrhea and four times the risk of developing Irritable Bowel Syndrome.

The medical records of personnel deployed in Operations Iraqi Freedom and Enduring Freedom indicate the fourth leading cause of their visits to Veterans Affairs medical centers was chronic gastrointestinal disorders. As many as 20 percent of these patients have conditions that have persisted for five years or longer after returning home.

It's not hard to understand the high incidence of this problem, considering the stress these soldiers are under and the less-than-sanitary conditions they're exposed to. What is hard to understand is the way these men and women are being treated.

Typical treatment focuses on the use of antibiotics to wipe out the offending bacteria. Patients are then switched to over-the-counter diarrhea medicine and bulking agents when the problem persists. Knowing what we know today, I'm amazed that probiotics aren't being used to correct and ultimately prevent such problems.

If you have a friend or loved one on overseas military duty, keep them supplied. New research continues to show that probiotics really are a gift that keeps on giving.

Using the details in Part I of this book, you'll be well on your way to building a solid foundation for digestive wellness. Eating a healthy diet, drinking pure water, effectively managing your stress, and creating an all-important bacterial balance in your bowels, will provide significant relief of your digestive discomforts all on their own.

And even if your particular condition requires further steps, you'll be starting those with the very best digestive system basics in place. Certainly, this effectively sets the stage for true digestive healing and long-term wellness.

In Part II of this book, I'll address the top digestive conditions affecting Americans today, and the safe, proven tools and techniques you can use to vanquish them and finally find lasting relief.

PART II

Action Plans for Specific Conditions

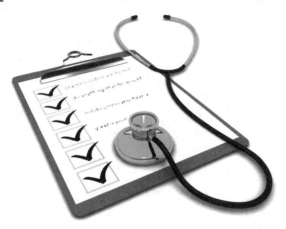

Now that you know the building blocks for creating a healthy digestive system foundation, let's next turn our attention to the six major digestive ailments that are inflicting so much misery on so many people. These include:

- Acid Reflux/GERD

- Ulcers

- IBS—Irritable Bowel Syndrome

- Food Allergies (including Celiac Disease)

- IBD—Inflammatory Bowel Disease (including Ulcerative Colitis and Crohn's Disease)

- Colorectal Cancer

Keep reading for details about these conditions and disorders, as well as an action plan addressing each—complete with dietary suggestions, nutrient recommendations, and techniques that have brought relief to others.

Acid Reflux/GERD

Acid reflux and gastroesophageal reflux disease (GERD) are really the same condition in which stomach acid escapes up through the top of the stomach and into the esophagus—primarily due to a malfunctioning or weak lower esophageal sphincter (LES).

As you'll recall from the earlier digestive system anatomy overview, the LES is a muscular band at the bottom of your esophagus, which opens to allow food to move from the esophagus to the stomach and then closes to keep food or stomach acid from backing up into the esophagus.

Your stomach has a protective coating of mucosa to protect against this acid, but your esophagus doesn't. So when stomach acid comes in contact with the tender esophageal tissue, it causes inflammation and a burning sensation—commonly referred to as heartburn. (For more details on heartburn, turn to page 98 in Part III of this book.)

Heartburn is often felt behind the breast bone in your chest, but can radiate from the rib cage to the neck. Chronic heartburn can cause regurgitation into the throat and mouth, along with a stinging sensation there, a sour taste in your mouth, and excessive salivation.

Although heartburn is the most common symptom of GERD, you can have GERD without heartburn. What you may experience instead are the often-overlooked symptoms of GERD. These include asthma symptoms, trouble swallowing, a dry cough, chronic hoarseness, laryngitis, persistent throat clearing, recurrent sore throat, and repeated ear and sinus infections.

? **Did You Know…**

An estimated 70% of asthma sufferers also have problems with acid reflux. The coughing and gagging that can occur when acid enters the esophagus often allows small amounts of acid to enter the airways, which results in an asthma attack.

People with asthma problems often enjoy dramatic improvements after they take steps to relieve their GERD.

A common burn

Statistics on the frequency of heartburn vary, but all confirm that it's a common condition. It's estimated that 15 million Americans have heartburn every day and more than 60 million feel the burn at least once a month.

If you have heartburn symptoms two to three times a week or more, you would be classified as suffering from GERD. Although this condition can affect people of all ages, statistics show that the risk increases with age—accelerating dramatically after age 40. Approximately 20 percent of the adult population in America is said to have GERD.

Drug chart: acid reflux/GERD

Drug Type—Alumiunum-Based Antacid

Brand Name	Generic Name	Potential Side Effects
Amphoget, Gaviscon, Maalox, Mylanta	N/A	Constipation, diarrhea, loss of appetite, mood swings, muscle weakness

Drug Type—Calcium-Based Antacid

Brand Name	Generic Name	Potential Side Effects
Alka-Mints, Caltrate, Rolaids, Tums	N/A	Chalky texture, unpleasant taste, constipation, loss of appetite, mood swings, muscle pain

Drug Type—Magnesium-Based Antacid

Brand Name	Generic Name	Potential Side Effects
Gaviscon, Gelusil, Maalox, Mylanta, Phillips' Milk of Magnesia	N/A	Chalky texture, dizziness, irregular heartbeat, loss of appetite, mood swings, muscle weakness

Drug Type—Sodium Bicarbonate-Based Antacid

Brand Name	Generic Name	Potential Side Effects
Alka-Seltzer, baking soda	N/A	Burping, feeling of fullness, frequent urge to urinate, mood swings, muscle pain, nausea, restlessness

Drug Type—H2 Histamine Blockers

Brand Name	Generic Name	Potential Side Effects
Tagamet, Pepcid, Axid, Zantac	cimetidine, famotidine, nizatidine, ranitidine	Rarely, may cause diarrhea, constipation, dizziness, anxiety, depression, drowsiness, sleeplessness, headache, irregular heartbeat, increased sweating, burning, itching, redness of skin, fever, confusion in ill or elderly people

Drug Type—Proton Pump Inhibitors

Brand Name	Generic Name	Potential Side Effects
Prevacid	lansoprazole	Rarely, may cause diarrhea, abdominal pain, nausea
Prilosec, Zegerid, Aciphex, Protonix, Nexium	omeprazole, rabeprazole, pantoprazole, esomeprazole	Rarely, may cause constipation, chest pain, headache, gas, rash, drowsiness

Amount Spent (over-the-counter antacids): $2 Billion—Source: AARP

Amount Spent (proton pump inhibitors): $14.1 Billion—Source: Nutrition Business Journal, 2009

Source: Adapted from, Harvard Medical School, *The Sensitive Gut Report* (Boston: Harvard Health Publications, 2010)

? Did You Know...

Logic would tell you that your stomach secretes most of its digestive acids with every meal, but that isn't the case. From 10 p.m. to 2 a.m., it secretes two to three times more acid than at any other time.

Some researchers believe this is part of a cleansing process that helps destroy residual pathogens. Regardless of why it happens, this night time acid production causes a great deal of distress for many people, particularly older adults.

Contributing factors

Although a weak LES is thought to be the primary cause of GERD, other factors can contribute to the problem. For instance, weak stomach muscles that don't contract and move food on to the small intestines in a timely manner can cause a backup of food and stomach acids into the esophagus. Also, increased abdominal pressure from weight gain or pregnancy can result in acid reflux and heartburn pain. Additionally, pregnancy hormones are thought to relax the LES and invite heartburn.

Traditional thinking points to a number of things that can aggravate your heartburn, including foods that increase gastric acid secretions, like spicy dishes, fried and high-fat foods, tomatoes and tomato-based products, citrus fruits, garlic, onions, and mints. Certain drinks, such as alcoholic beverages, caffeinated coffee and tea, carbonated drinks, and even milk; stressful emotions; and even particular body positions, like reclining in bed or bending over at the waist.

And now, new data has pointed to some other—often surprising—risk factors for acid reflux. Specifically, researchers in Norway evaluated study surveys comparing 3,153 individuals who reported problems with severe heartburn or regurgitation to 40,210 people without acid reflux symptoms.

They discovered that someone who smokes has almost double the risk of having acid reflux, which isn't a big surprise since smoking is associated with other poor health habits, such as the consumption of fried and fatty foods. More surprising was the finding that individuals who routinely added salt to their meals also had almost twice the risk of experiencing acid reflux.

Researchers also discovered that those who consumed coffee and high-fiber foods, and who exercised frequently, had a significantly lower incidence of acid reflux. Although the coffee finding contradicts conventional wisdom about avoiding caffeinated foods if you suffer from acid reflux, the greatest impact came from high-fiber diets. Researchers found that a fiber-rich diet could cut the incidence of reflux by almost half.[7]

? Did You Know...

A surprising symptom of chronic GERD is dental decay caused by the caustic action of stomach acid on your tooth enamel.

Chewing gum sweetened with xylitol instead of with sugar or an artificial sweetener will help protect your teeth by increasing saliva to wash away errant acids. And xylitol has been shown in scientific studies to help prevent tooth decay by inhibiting the action of certain bacteria that ferment in your mouth and cause cavities.

Complications of chronic GERD

Because digestive juices created in the stomach are very caustic, continued exposure to them in the esophagus and throat—where there is an insufficient protective mucus shield—can lead to other, more serious health concerns.

One of these conditions is *reflux esophagitis*. This is when stomach acids not only cause inflammation in the esophagus, but actually create areas of erosion in its mucus lining. People with esophagitis often experience more intense burning than the traditional discomfort of heartburn, with pain radiating into the neck, jaw, and even to the ears. At times the pain is so severe that it's mistaken for a heart attack. Also, the inflammation in the esophagus can cause difficulty swallowing, sensitivity to hot beverages, a persistent cough, nausea, and even bleeding.

Another condition resulting from constant exposure to stomach acids is *Barrett's esophagus*. This is when protective cells, like those normally found in the small intestine, begin to replace the normal cells lining the esophagus.

There are few symptoms of Barrett's esophagus, other than the same ones that carry over from GERD. People at greatest risk for the condition are older white males, particularly those who have higher incomes and have suffered with GERD for many years.

A number of studies have shown that having Barrett's esophagus increases your risk of esophageal cancer by up to 10 times, and the risk of adenocarcinoma (cancerous changes that are limited to the epithelial layer of a structure) by a factor of nearly 30.[8]

Although there aren't many new cases of esophageal cancer annually, the condition is particularly deadly, and the incidence is rising. The National Cancer Institute estimates that in 2007 there were about 15,500 new cases of esophageal cancer, and nearly 14,000 deaths. The annual incidence has increased by 570 percent over the last 25 years.

What <u>NOT</u> to do if you have acid reflux or GERD

Before I get into the specifics of what you should do to cool the fires of acid reflux and GERD, let me tell you what you shouldn't do…and that's submit blindly to the unrelenting hype of Big Pharma.

If you're diagnosed with GERD, chances are your doctor will prescribe a drug to "treat" it. This is an all-too-common approach in our modern medical world—masking symptoms instead of addressing underlying causes.

Drug company sales statistics speak volumes about this growing problem. The second best-selling prescription pharmaceutical in the United States in 2008 (the latest year with complete data available) was Nexium—a drug used to address GERD.

This widely prescribed drug (over 28 million prescriptions were written for it in 2008 alone) is extraordinarily expensive, costing $240 per month. Bad for your wallet, but great for AstraZeneca, the pharmaceutical company that produces the famous "purple pill." It pulled in an eye-popping 4.8 billion dollars in sales, which was second only to the cholesterol-lowering blockbuster drug, Lipitor. Prevacid, another drug prescribed for GERD, took fifth place, with 3.3 billion in sales.[9]

These drugs belong to a class known as proton pump inhibitors (PPIs), which block an enzyme in your stomach that produces acid. This, in turn, is supposed to prevent and heal ulcers in the stomach, esophagus, and duodenum.

Another class of prescription drugs for acid reflux is H_2 histamine blockers, like Zantac, Pepcid, and Tagamet. These work to block certain histamine receptors in the digestive tract that signal the release of digestive acids.

No cure...but more problems

While these drugs may provide symptomatic relief, they offer no cure. And, thanks to some of the most aggressive marketing campaigns in history, they are excessively prescribed and often taken long term. This, rather than healing your digestive system, can have devastating effects.

As ironic as it sounds, the last thing you want to do when you suffer from acid reflux is to reduce the production or acidity of your gastric juices. To understand why, consider the reason your body produces these acids in the first place.

Specialized cells in your stomach secrete acid in response to the presence of food or drink, and this acid is absolutely necessary for proper digestion. So, anything that interferes with acidity also interferes with digestion.

As poorly digested food particles make their way into the rest of your digestive tract, they can pass through your intestinal walls. There, they are identified as foreign material and your body mounts an allergic immune response, with troubling consequences for your digestive system and overall health.

Also, proper acid levels are needed to absorb certain vitamins and minerals, including vitamin B12 and calcium.

? **Did You Know...**

Every third TV commercial is a drug advertisement. By the time the average child reaches 18, he or she has seen 20,000 hours of drug commercials such as "Plop-plop, fizz-fizz, oh what a relief it is!"

Even those innocent antacids can spell T-R-O-U-B-L-E

Statistics show that people spend nearly 2 billion dollars a year on over-the-counter antacids. And, again, while these medicines can provide short-term relief for heartburn symptoms, they are far from worry-free.

Recent research has shown that antacids can cause significant changes in your urine. Specifically, antacids cause your urine to become more alkaline when it should be slightly acidic. If your urine stays too alkaline, an overgrowth of *E. coli* bacteria can result, leading to urinary tract infections.

Also, overuse of certain antacids could contribute to kidney stone formation. Calcium-based antacids, like Rolaids, Tums, Caltrate, and Alka-Mints add calcium to the blood, but also neutralize acid. Together, this can promote stone formation.

(Continued on page 34...)

A Surprising Cause of Much Reflux Suffering

There is a physical condition of the stomach that can cause many GERD-type symptoms—including heartburn, stomach acid backing up into the throat, and a sour stomach—and it's called a hiatal hernia. This condition is surprisingly common. I've seen them in people of all ages. Studies have shown that 32 percent of people over 50 and 89 percent of those over 90 have them!

What is a hiatal hernia?

Your diaphragm is a large dome-shaped muscle that separates the organs in the top part of your chest from your stomach and other digestive organs in the bottom half. In the back part of this muscle there is a button-shaped hole that allows your esophagus to go from your throat to your stomach. Sometimes this hole gets enlarged and the stomach can worm its way up into the hole. This is a hiatal hernia.

A hiatal hernia can change the angle of the esophagus where it joins the stomach, weaken ligaments around this juncture, and impair the LES from sealing stomach acids off from the esophagus.

How to test for a hiatal hernia

This is not a foolproof test, but a good initial screening for a hiatal hernia. Simply take a deep breath and hold it for 40 seconds. If you can't hold your breath for that long, and there are no other problems, it's possible you have a hiatal hernia.

What to do for a hiatal hernia

If you suspect you have a hiatal hernia, there are two ways you can try to reverse it on your own.

The first way:

Drink a glass of room temperature or slightly warm water first thing in the morning when you get out of bed. (No coffee, tea, juice, or cold water… just warm water.)

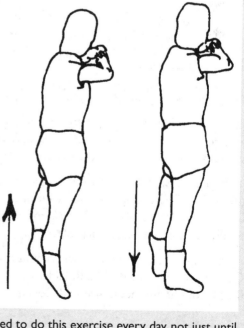

Then stand straight with your feet about hip distance apart. Bring your arms straight out to your sides and then bend your elbows so your hands are touching your chest. Stand on your toes as high as possible, and then drop so that you get a pretty good jolt. (See illustration.) Do this about 10 times in a row.

Then, while standing with your arms up, pant short, quick breaths for 10 to 15 seconds. That's it! Note: You'll need to do this exercise every day, not just until everything feels normal.

(Continued on next page…)

(Continued from page 32...)

Aluminum-based antacids, like Maalox, Mylanta, and Gaviscon, could cause a build-up of aluminum in your blood. Although you may only absorb a fraction of the amount you ingest, depending on the brand you use and how often you take them, you could be exposing yourself to as much as 3 grams or more of inorganic aluminum daily.

We already know that high amounts of aluminum in drinking water and food can cause nerve damage and memory loss. Aluminum buildup is also associated with bone demineralization or weakening and many of the same horrors associated with osteoporosis.

Furthermore, like their more powerful prescription cousins, antacids reduce hydrochloric acid levels in the stomach, which exacerbates the natural decline of hydrochloric acid with age. A person's stomach at age 50 only releases 15 percent of the amount of acid it released at age 25. And even more alarming, 35 percent of all individuals over 65 don't produce any hydrochloric acid at all! This is troubling because your stomach needs high hydrochloric acid levels in order to properly digest certain nutrients, like calcium, iron, and protein.

Temporary heartburn relief from antacids is simply not worth all of these health risks. Please turn the page for your action plan for acid reflux/GERD.

⟫ Your Action Plan for Acid Reflux/GERD ⟫

There are safe, proven, natural tools and techniques that you can use to ease symptoms and—more importantly—address the root causes of reflux and GERD. I've listed them here as an "action plan" for you to follow.

1. **Eat a healthy, low-fat diet.** A healthful diet, like the one I outlined for you in Part I of this book, is easy on your digestive system and filled with nutrients to support healthy digestive function. Make a conscious effort to also steer clear of the most common reflux "trigger foods" such as spicy dishes, fried and high-fat foods, tomatoes and tomato-based products, citrus fruits, garlic, onions, mints, alcoholic beverages, caffeinated coffee and tea, carbonated drinks, and milk. Also, avoid excess salt. Instead, experiment with healthful herbs and spices to enhance the flavor of your food.

   It's also a good idea to eat smaller meals spread throughout the day, to eat slowly and chew thoroughly, and never eat if you're not hungry or if you're upset. After eating, wait at least an hour before exercising, and at least 3 hours before lying down.

   As a bonus, your healthy eating habits should help you lose excess pounds, which helps reduce the pressure on your abdomen that can cause acid reflux and contribute to digestive discomfort.

2. **Drink at least 8–10 eight-ounce glasses of pure, clean water every day.** This is good advice for healthy digestion and overall wellness, but is especially important if you suffer from acid reflux because it helps to rinse away stray stomach acid.

   Drink one to two glasses of water when you get up in the morning and a half hour before meals. And take your nutritional supplements at meal times with tall glasses of water.

3. **Stop smoking.** This bad habit has been shown in studies to increase your risk of acid reflux, as well as a plethora of other health problems.

4. **Avoid tight-fitting clothing** that can constrict your abdomen.

5. **Chew gum.** This simple strategy not only helps prevent the dental decay that can come with chronic reflux, but also helps to soothe the esophagus and wash digestive acids back down into the stomach where they belong.

6. **Try hydrochloric acid.** If you are over 50 years of age, a natural decline in your hydrochloric acid production may be contributing to acid reflux, in which case supplementation can help.

   I always recommend betaine hydrochloride, which you can get at health food stores. One really important point to remember is to take one or two tablets after you eat, not before or during your meal. You want your stomach to produce and secrete as much acid as it can before adding the additional acid.

7. **Add digestive enzymes.** In addition to hydrochloric acid, there are dozens of digestive enzymes on the market that can help re-acidify your intestinal tract improve your overall digestive capabilities, and relieve your reflux symptoms.

   A good product will include acids and enzymes similar to those produced by the stomach, like pepsin and betaine hydrochloride. It should also include enzymes commonly produced by the pancreas and those present in the bile from the gallbladder.

   If you can't find a good digestive enzyme product at a health food store, call Progressive Laboratories at 1-800-527-9512 or visit their website for more information, *progressivelabs.com*. They sell an excellent product called Digestin #987. Just follow the directions on the bottle.

8. **Take deglycyrrhizinated licorice (DGL).** This herbal extract promotes your gastrointestinal tract's natural defense mechanisms, increases production of protective mucosal cells, and helps reduce inflammation.

   DGL has a long history of medicinal use and research, and I've seen it help people with a variety of GERD symptoms, including chronic heartburn, persistent cough, asthma-like symptoms, and a hiatal hernia (see the box on pages 33–34 for more details on this.)

   The suggested dose of DGL is two tablets, chewed about 20 minutes before meals, three times a day. Use only chewable DGL—it must be mixed with saliva in order to be effective. Unlike regular licorice, DGL will not cause water retention, raise blood pressure, or lower testosterone levels. This supplement, which is also beneficial for ulcers and canker sores, can be found in most health food stores.

9. **Consider other herbal remedies to soothe your digestive tract, including chamomile and ginger.** Enjoying a cup of chamomile tea can help you relax, de-stress, and calm an irritated stomach.

   Ginger root powder is well known for its effectiveness against pain and motion sickness, but it can also be useful for soothing symptoms of acid reflux. Use a teaspoon of freshly grated root each day. If that's not possible or you find it inconvenient, then try taking 1,000 mg (approximately ¼ teaspoon) of the ginger root powder in either capsules or in bulk powder form.

If your reflux symptoms are worse at night, also consider these steps…

10. **Raise the head of your bed by 4–6 inches.** Make sure you do this by inserting blocks, bricks, or a wedge made specifically for this purpose and available at most medical supply stores, under your mattress…and not by adding pillows under your head. Additional pillows cause your body to bend at the waist near your stomach and can actually aggravate nighttime reflux symptoms.

11. Keep a glass of water by your bed. If you experience any uncomfortable burning sensations that wake you up, you can take a quick sip to wash stray acids back into your stomach.

• *Track Your Success!* •

To track your success with this Action Plan, I highly recommend that you record the exact steps you're taking to address your acid reflux or GERD each day, as well as the symptoms you are experiencing at the time, and how you are feeling emotionally.

Putting these details on paper is an excellent way to see what works for you. It's also a great way to document the improvements you're experiencing and just how far you've come using safe, natural solutions to your digestive problem.

Turn to pages 135–136 for sample pages that makes tracking this information simple. Use these pages as your master copy and photocopy more pages to fill in with your details.

Ulcers

Digestive ulcers, also known as peptic ulcers, are places where the protective coating of mucus has been eroded away from the lining of your stomach or upper digestive tract. The most common type is the duodenal ulcer, which occurs in the first 12 inches of the small intestine, just beyond the stomach. Ulcers that form in the stomach are called gastric ulcers. Ulcers can also form in the esophagus, and these are called esophageal ulcers.

The discomfort you experience with a peptic ulcer is similar to that of heartburn—burning or gnawing feeling. Only you're likely to feel this in your upper abdomen instead of behind your breastbone. The feeling is usually intermittent, lasting between 30 minutes to 3 hours, and it's often mistaken for heartburn, indigestion, or even hunger.

Some people experience ulcer pain right after eating, but others don't have pain until hours later. This may be a factor of where the ulcer is located. Duodenal ulcers are often relieved by food, while gastric ulcers can be aggravated by it. Quite often ulcer pain is more intense overnight, perhaps because this is when stomach acid production is at its peak and has greater potential to irritate ulcerated areas in the stomach or small intestine.

Other symptoms of a peptic ulcer are bloating, gas and feelings of abdominal fullness, loss of appetite, and unexpected weight loss. Rare, but dangerous complications of peptic ulcers include gastric obstruction from inflammation and scarring; perforation of the GI wall, leading to the leakage of stomach or intestine contents into the abdominal cavity; and penetration, where the ulcer spreads to other organs, such as the pancreas and liver.

Symptoms of these more advanced ulcer conditions include persistent nausea, repeated vomiting, vomiting of blood, feeling cold and clammy, feeling dizzy or unusually weak, blood in your stools, and sudden severe pain in the abdomen.

A pain shared by many

It's estimated that about 20 million Americans develop at least one ulcer during their lifetime and that this condition affects 4–5 million Americans each year. Furthermore, each year approximately 40,000 Americans resort to surgery in a desperate bid to end their ulcer pain. And about 6,000 Americans die of stomach ulcer–related complications every year.

Although ulcers can develop at any age, they are rare in children and uncommon in teenagers. Duodenal ulcers usually first appear

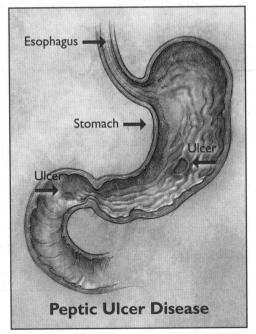

Esophagus

Stomach

Ulcer

Ulcer

Peptic Ulcer Disease

(Continued on page 41...)

PART II

Drug chart: ulcers

Drug Type—Antibiotics

Brand Name	Generic Name	Potential Side Effects
Flagyl, Sumycin, Biaxin, Amoxil	metronidazole, tetracycline, clarithromycin, amoxicillin	Nausea, vomiting, diarrhea, dry mouth, upset stomach, indigestion, hepatotoxicity, intestinal *Candida* infection, antibiotic colitis, *C difficile* infection, gut dysbiosis

Drug Type—H2 Blockers

Brand Name	Generic Name	Potential Side Effects
Tagamet, Zantac, Pepcid, Axid	cimetidine, ranitidine, famotidine, nizatidine	Breast enlargement in men (especially with Tagamet), constipation, diarrhea, nausea or vomiting, dizziness, drowsiness, headache, irritated or runny nose, pain, rash, sore throat, weakness

Drug Type—Proton Pump Inhibitors

Brand Name	Generic Name	Potential Side Effects
Prevacid	lansoprazole	Rarely, may cause diarrhea, abdominal pain, nausea
Prilosec, Zegerid, Aciphex, Protonix, Nexium	omeprazole, rabeprazole, pantaprazole, esomeprazole	Rarely, may cause constipation, chest pain, headache, gas, rash, drowsiness

Drug Type—Stomach Lining Protectors

Brand Name	Generic Name	Potential Side Effects
Pepto-Bismol	bismuth subsalicylate	Dark tongue, grayish-black stools. Excessive doses may cause anxiety, constipation, dizziness

Drug Type—Aluminum-Based Antacid

Brand Name	Generic Name	Potential Side Effects
Amphoget, Gaviscon, Maalox, Mylanta	N/A	Constipation, diarrhea, loss of appetite, mood swings, muscle weakness

Drug Type—Calcium-Based Antacid

Brand Name	Generic Name	Potential Side Effects
Alka-Mints, Caltrate, Rolaids, Tums	N/A	Chalky texture, unpleasant taste, constipation, loss of appetite, mood swings, muscle pain

Drug Type—Magnesium-Based Antacid

Brand Name	Generic Name	Potential Side Effects
Gaviscon, Gelusil, Maalox, Mylanta, Phillips' Milk of Magnesia	N/A	Chalky texture, dizziness, irregular heartbeat, loss of appetite, mood swings, muscle weakness

Drug Type—Sodium Bicarbonate-Based Antacid

Brand Name	Generic Name	Potential Side Effects
Alka-Seltzer	N/A	Burping, feeling of fullness, frequent urge to urinate, mood swings, muscle pain, nausea, restlessness

Drug chart: ulcers continued...

Drug Type—H2 Histamine Blockers

Brand Name	Generic Name	Potential Side Effects
Tagamet, Pepcid, Axid, Zantac	cimetidine, famotidine, nizatidine, ranitidine	Rarely, may cause diarrhea, constipation, dizziness, anxiety, depression, drowsiness, sleeplessness, headache, irregular heartbeat, increased sweating, burning, itching, redness of skin, fever, confusion in ill or elderly people

Drug Type—Proton Pump Inhibitors

Brand Name	Generic Name	Potential Side Effects
Prevacid	lansoprazole	Rarely, may cause diarrhea, abdominal pain, nausea
Prilosec, Zegerid, Aciphex, Protonix, Nexium	omeprazole, rabeprazole, pantoprazole, esomeprazole	Rarely, may cause constipation, chest pain, headache, gas, rash, drowsiness

Drug Type—Antispasmodics

Brand Name	Generic Name	Potential Side Effects
Acro-Lase Plus	atropine with hyoscyamine and phenobarbital	Dry mouth, difficulty urinating or urinary retention, blurred vision, rapid heartbeat, increased ocular tension, headache, nervousness. drowsiness. Antispasmodics that contain phenobarbital may cause sedation, drowsiness, or, rarely, agitation
Donnatal	atropine with hyoscyamine, phenobarbital, and scopolamine	
Bentyl	dycyclomine	
Levsin	hyoscyamine	

Drug Type—Antidiarrheal Agents

Brand Name	Generic Name	Potential Side Effects
Lomotil	diphenoxylate and atropine	Abdominal discomfort, constipation; less frequently, may cause blurred vision, urinary discomfort, dry mouth or skin, rapid heartbeat, restlessness, or warm, flushed skin
Imodium, Imodium A-D	loperamide	Abdominal discomfort, constipation; less frequently, may cause drowsiness, dizziness, dry mouth, nausea, vomiting, rash

Drug Type—Laxatives

Brand Name	Generic Name	Potential Side Effects
Colace, Surfak	docusate	Stomach or intestinal cramps, stomach upset, throat irritation
Kondremul Lubricant and Fleet	mineral oil	May cause deficiencies of fat-soluble vitamins if used regularly; can cause lung damage if accidentally inhaled
MiraLAX	polyethylene glycol	Upset stomach, bloating, cramping, gas
Correctol, Dulcolax, Fleet,	bisacodyl	Stomach cramps, upset stomach, diarrhea, stomach and intestinal irritation, faintness, irritation or burning in the rectum (from suppositories)
Purge, Fleet	castor oil	Diarrhea, upset stomach, vomiting, irritation, stomach cramping

PART II

(Continued on next page...)

Drug chart: ulcers continued...		
Ex-Lax, Fletcher's Castoria, Senokot,	senna	Diarrhea, upset stomach, vomiting, irritation, stomach cramping, pseudomelanosis coli
Drug Type—SSRIs		
Brand Name	**Generic Name**	**Potential Side Effects**
Celexa	citalopram	Upset stomach, diarrhea, vomiting, stomach pain, drowsiness, excessive tiredness, tremors, excitement, nervousness, difficulty falling or staying asleep, muscle or joint pain, dry mouth, excessive sweating, changes in sex drive or ability, loss of appetite
Prozac	fluoxetine	Rash, headache, dizziness, insomnia, anxiety, drowsiness, excessive sweating, nausea, diarrhea, bronchitis, weight loss, painful menstruation, sexual dysfunction, urinary tract infection, chills, muscle or joint pain, back pain
Paxil	paroxetine	Pain, bodily discomfort, hypertension, sudden loss of strength, rapid heartbeat, itching, nausea, vomiting, weight gain or loss, central nervous system stimulation, depression, vertigo, cough
Zoloft	sertraline	Nausea, trouble sleeping, diarrhea, dry mouth, sexual dysfunction, drowsiness, tremor, indigestion, increased sweating, increased irritability or anxiety, decreased appetite
Drug Type—Serotonin Regulators		
Brand Name	**Generic Name**	**Potential Side Effects**
Lotronex	alosetron	Constipation; in rare cases, may cause diarrhea and intestinal bleeding
Zelnorm	tegaserod	Diarrhea, stomach pain, increased risk of heart attack, stroke, and unstable angina
Drug Type—Tricyclic Antidepressants		
Brand Name	**Generic Name**	**Potential Side Effects**
Elavil, Endep	amitriptyline	Dizziness, dry mouth, blurred vision, drowsiness, constipation, urinary retention, hypotension, cardiac arrhythmia
Norpramine	desipramine	
Pamelor	nortriptyline	

Source: Adapted from, Harvard Medical School, *The Sensitive Gut Report* (Boston: Harvard Health Publications, 2010)

(Continued from page 38...)

between the ages of 30 and 50, and are more common in men than women. Gastric ulcers are more likely to develop in people over age 60, and are more common in women than men.

Suspected causes

For many years, it was thought that peptic ulcers were caused by spicy foods and stress, but research has since debunked these theories. It's worth noting, however, that high-fat diets and stress, which can both hinder healthy digestion, could certainly exacerbate an ulcer.

Smoking

Another unhealthy lifestyle factor—smoking—has been shown to have a more direct link to ulcers. Research has shown that smoking increases the chance of getting an ulcer, slows the healing process of existing ulcers, and can make ulcers more likely to recur.

Some studies indicate that smoking impairs the body's ability to neutralize stomach acid once it reaches your duodenum, which would increase the risk of ulcers in this part of your digestive tract. Other studies suggest that cigarette smoking may increase the amount of acid secreted by the stomach over time, which could complicate healing and intensify the pain of gastric ulcers.[10]

NSAIDs

More recently, NSAIDs—including aspirin, ibuprofen, naproxen, ketoprofen, and many arthritis drugs—have been identified as a major cause of peptic ulcers. These powerful anti-inflammatory drugs work to decrease inflammation and pain by inhibiting the body's production of prostaglandins.

Unfortunately, certain prostaglandins also play an important role in maintaining the protective lining in your stomach, which guards against the corrosive effects of stomach acid. Therefore, by inhibiting prostaglandin production, NSAIDs also put the health of your stomach lining at risk and taking these drugs—especially if you take them long term—increases your chances of developing peptic ulcers.

? Did You Know…

In addition to increasing your risk of developing ulcers and gastrointestinal bleeding, overuse of NSAIDs can increase the permeability of your entire gastrointestinal tract. And when this happens, larger proteins, bacteria, and toxins are able to enter your bloodstream, resulting in allergic reactions, increased stress to the immune system, and the spread of toxins throughout your body.

It's estimated that up to 50 percent of patients can't tolerate NSAID treatment because of its gastrointestinal side effects. And approximately 15 percent of patients on long-term NSAID treatment develop peptic ulcers. Furthermore, approximately 100,000 Americans are hospitalized each year, and between 15,000 and 20,000 Americans die each year, from ulcers and gastrointestinal bleeding linked to NSAID use.

People at greatest risk for developing serious GI complications with NSAID use are those who have rheumatoid arthritis, take blood thinners or cortisone medications, have heart disease, or are elderly.[11]

Although long-term NSAID use has been a known risk factor of ulcers for some time, a new "smoking gun" has recently materialized—the *Helicobacter pylori* (*H. pylori*) bacteria.

Helicobacter pylori bacteria

In the early 1980s, researchers identified *H. pylori* as a major factor in the development of peptic ulcers. This corkscrew-shaped pathogen literally twists its way through the protective mucus lining of the gastrointestinal tract and attaches itself to the walls of your stomach or small intestine.

Research suggests that almost 90 percent of people with duodenal ulcers and up to 85 percent of those with gastric ulcers harbor the *H. pylori* bacteria. Unfortunately, in the typical "take no prisoners" style of conventional medicine, the treatment of choice for ulcers suddenly became a 2– to 3–week course of strong antibiotics, with the goal of totally eliminating the offending bacteria from the body.

Unfortunately, antibiotics do not discriminate in the bacteria that they vanquish. They take the good with the bad and cause a total upset of the delicate bacterial balance throughout your digestive tract.

Like thousands of other strains of bacteria in our environment, *H. pylori* doesn't seem to cause problems when its numbers remain in balance with other bacterial flora. In fact, researchers from Stanford University School of Medicine recently reported that individuals with *H. pylori* in their system have a 72 percent *lower* risk of developing esophageal cancer than individuals without the bacterium.

This is because *H. pylori* has been shown to lower the acid-secreting ability of the stomach, which appears to provide a protective effect against acid erosion of the esophagus and small intestine. Many individuals begin to experience acid reflux and GERD when *H. pylori* is totally eliminated from the body. Continued damage and destruction to the tissues can then lead to esophageal cancer.

Similar studies have questioned the use of a medical procedure called "eradication therapy," wherein antibiotics are used to wipe out or "cure" an *H. pylori* infection. For instance, in one research study, when 87 patients with ulcers were given antibiotics and followed for a year, 21 percent of them developed inflammation of the esophagus, and 37 percent showed evidence of GERD, compared with only 8 percent in the non-antibiotic group.[12]

Some authorities now believe that the widespread use of antibiotics and the reduction in gastrointestinal *H. pylori* may be why the incidence of esophageal adenocarcinoma has been increasing faster than any other cancer in the U.S. and parts of Europe over the last 20 to 30 years.[13]

? Did You Know...

Antibiotics—some of the most common medicines now prescribed for peptic ulcers—are possibly the worst offenders known for causing stomach upset. Antibiotics particularly noted for causing nausea and indigestion are erythromycin, tetracycline, and trimethoprim-sulfamethoxazole.

Diagnosing an ulcer

Because symptoms of an ulcer can vary quite widely from individual to individual, your doctor may suggest testing to confirm that you do have an ulcer, identify where it is in your GI tract, and get a better idea of how advanced the ulcer is.

Testing can include an upper GI series, where you drink a chalky barium contrast dye, followed by x-rays of your esophagus, stomach, and duodenum. The barium dye helps to make these organs more visible on the x-rays.

Another, more invasive test is the endoscopy, where a small, flexible tube with a camera and surgical tools on the end is threaded through your mouth and into your esophagus, stomach, and duodenum. The camera gives your doctor a look at these organs and the surgical tools can be used to take biopsy samples, if necessary, or to cauterize a bleeding ulcer.

I don't recommend these tests unless your symptoms indicate complications from an advanced ulcer, where surgery to stop bleeding may be necessary. Otherwise, the effort, expense, and risks of the procedures outweigh the benefit of additional information you would gain. And, the steps I recommend for healing your ulcers will improve your GI health regardless of where your ulcer happens to be.

Also be aware that doctors who buy into the *H. pylori* blame game for ulcers often suggest testing your blood, breath, stool, and stomach tissue to see if the bacteria is present. And, if it is, you'll most certainly be given a prescription for antibiotics.

But, the fact of the matter is that *H. pylori* resides in 50 percent of the world's population—most of whom don't have trouble with ulcers. Furthermore, *H. pylori* has been shown to have specific health benefits, if it's in proper balance with other gastrointestinal bacteria.

So, testing for *H. pylori* and then "treating" it with antibiotics doesn't make a shred of sense to me. It only serves to disrupt the balance of bacterial flora in your digestive tract and set the stage for other digestive and immune system problems.

Please turn the page for your action plan for ulcers.

⫸ Your Action Plan for Ulcers ⫸

As with acid reflux and GERD, there are a number of safe, effective tools and techniques you can use to get to the root of your ulcer problem by restoring health to the lining of your esophagus, stomach, and duodenum. And there are steps you can take—including a number of important lifestyle changes—that will significantly reduce the risk of ulcer recurrence.

1. **Eat healthful foods in a mindful way.** As with all digestive health issues, eating a healthy, low-fat, nutrient-dense diet is imperative. Beyond basic steps, you should also make sure to avoid any foods that you find cause irritation, heartburn, and stomach upset. And stay away from alcohol, which increases the production of stomach acid and can irritate an ulcer and worsen symptoms.

   Also, make a point to eat smaller, more frequent meals. This keeps your stomach from getting too full and creating unwanted gastric pressure, which can lead to irritation.

   Finally, don't eat anything for at least 3 hours before going to bed. Lying down with a full stomach can increase your chances of reflux and irritation to your esophagus.

2. **Don't smoke.** Smoking stimulates the production of stomach acid. It can also delay the healing of ulcers, and has been linked to a recurrence of ulcers.

3. **Avoid NSAIDs.** Overuse of these powerful anti-inflammatory drugs can compromise the protective lining in your stomach and put you at risk for ulcers.

4. **Balance the bacterial flora in your bowel with probiotics.** A diet rich in naturally fermented foods and homemade yogurt will help to naturally seed your digestion system with healthy probiotics and balance the bacterial flora in your bowels. Taking a quality probiotic supplement daily will also do this.

   Working to restore balance in your body as a means to resolve ulcers is a much more reasonable, safe, and gentle solution than to wipe out good and bad bacteria with powerful antibiotics, which seems to be the preferred methodology in conventional medical circles these days.

5. **Take deglycyrrhizinated licorice.** DGL enhances normal defense mechanisms that prevent ulcer formation. DGL increases the number of mucosal cells, thus increasing the amount of protective mucus that covers the GI tract cells. It also improves the quality of mucus production, seems to increase the lifespan of the intestinal cells, and enhances the microcirculation of blood through the GI tract lining.

   This form of licorice outperformed the prescription ulcer drug Tagamet and antacids in a study of people with chronic duodenal ulcers. Endoscopies revealed that the DGL group had 77% early improvement, versus 60% for those on Tagamet. At 12 weeks, the relapse rate with DGL was 8.2%, compared to 12.9% for the Tagamet group and 16.4% for the antacids.

Treating GI problems with DGL has no side effects, and is without a doubt safer than conventional medications. This remedy is sold in a chewable tablet because DGL needs saliva for activation. If you have an ulcer, chew three or four tablets three times daily, about 20 minutes before a meal, and again at bedtime. For prevention of ulcers and general improvement and maintenance of the gastrointestinal tract, two tablets two or three times daily before meals should suffice.

6. **Soothe your stomach with aloe vera.** This thick-leafed succulent is most well known as a topical remedy for burns and insect bites. But aloe is also beneficial for your GI tract. It enhances the digestion and absorption of food and reduces bacterial putrefaction in the gut.

Since the aloe plant is over 99.5% water, a product which claims to be "100% aloe vera juice" may indeed have only 0.5% of the active compounds. Concentrates—the stronger, the better—of the whole leaf are your best value. For ulcers, I recommend up to eight ounces a day of a concentrated aloe product in divided doses mixed with water. Look for Aloe Life, Aloe Master, Lily of the Desert, and Aloe Ace brands of aloe vera concentrates in health food stores.

7. **Eat more hot peppers.** Contrary to what many say, eating chili peppers doesn't cause ulcers. In fact, peppers have been shown to trigger mechanisms that actually protect the lining of the stomach.

Studies in Hungary have found that consumption of capsaicin, the active component of chili peppers, actually decreased the acid output of the stomach, while at the same time increasing protective secretions.

Capsaicin was also particularly effective at protecting the stomach from ulcerations caused by alcohol and NSAIDs. These drugs cause injury to the protective mucosal lining of the stomach, which can result in bleeding. Capsaicin reduced the amount of NSAID-induced bleeding dramatically.[14] Similar studies in Singapore revealed that eating the chili peppers reduced the risk of developing gastric ulcers by 53 percent.[15]

8. **Try a little honey.** Honey is a natural substance that has been used for hundreds of years in other countries to treat burns, wounds, sores, and a variety of other ailments. Honey works to heal ulcers through an enzyme it contains called glucose oxidase. This enzyme produces hydrogen peroxide, which works to kill harmful bacteria.

Honey is also known to reduce swelling around a wound through anti-inflammatory action, increase local circulation to a wound, and stimulate re-growth of damaged tissue, all of which promote a healing environment for ulcerated areas of your digestive tract.

The key to successful treatment is using natural, unprocessed honey. I recommend Manuka honey from New Zealand, which is available in nearly any health food store. Start with two tablespoons a day until your ulcer problem has eased. Then one tablespoon daily should be enough.

9. **Go bananas.** The sitoindosides in dried, unripe bananas increase mucus in the digestive tract, which provides a strong protective coating. Bananas also contain water-soluble polysaccharides, the same compounds found in the anti-ulcer prescription drug, Carafate.

   Unripe, whole, sweet bananas will have some effect, but you'll get the best results with banana powder. To make it on your own, peel the bananas and cut them into thin slices. Put the slices in the sun, an oven, or a food dehydrator, and dry them slowly. When dry, grind them into a fine powder. Mix two tablespoons of the powder with one tablespoon of honey. Take this mixture three times a day—mid-morning, mid-afternoon, and at bedtime.

10. **Consider vitamin E supplements.** Doctors at the Kiev Medical Institute reported that 300 mg of vitamin E daily effectively treated peptic ulcers of 28 patients. This dosage relieved ulcers in four to six days for the subject group given vitamin E, while it took seven to ten days for those given conventional medication. Patients taking vitamin E also had increased protein repair in their intestinal linings and gained from 1.5 to 3 kg during the study, while the controls did not gain any weight.[16]

11. **Maintain your melatonin.** One cause of ulcers rarely mentioned is low melatonin levels. The trigger for melatonin production in the pineal gland is low light levels. As our society stays up later, uses artificial lighting far into the night, and gets less sleep, our bodies obviously produce less melatonin. The use of NSAIDs and alcohol also impair melatonin production.

    Decreased melatonin production has been linked to increased rates of cancer, poor immune system function, and several other problems, including an increased incidence of ulcers.

    If you have a chronic ulcer problem, it's highly possible your production of melatonin is below normal. Animal studies have shown that increasing melatonin levels by even small amounts can have a dramatic effect in both healing and preventing stress-induced ulcers. I recommend 2–3 grams of melatonin daily, taken at bedtime.[17]

• • • • • • • • • • • • • • • • • Track Your Success! •

To track your success with this Action Plan, I highly recommend that you record the exact steps you're taking to address your ulcers each day, as well as the symptoms you are experiencing at the time, and how you are feeling emotionally.

Putting these details on paper is an excellent way to see what works for you. It's also a great way to document the improvements you're experiencing and just how far you've come using safe, natural solutions to your digestive problem.

Turn to pages 135–136 for sample pages that makes tracking this information simple. Use these pages as your master copy and photocopy more pages to fill in with your details.

Irritable Bowel Syndrome

Irritable bowel syndrome (IBS) is known by many names—functional bowel disease, spastic colon, spastic bowel, nervous indigestion, mucus colitis, and intestinal neurosis. But, regardless of its moniker, it's the most frequently diagnosed gastrointestinal condition in the United States.

In fact, between 30 percent and 50 percent of all referrals to gastroenterologists are because of IBS and it's estimated that as many as 35 million people have IBS in this country alone.[18] If you're one of them, you undoubtedly know how debilitating this condition can be.

Women seem to suffer from the problem more than men. This could be because the hormone fluctuations of menstruation, pregnancy, and menopause can all impact a woman's digestive tract and trigger bloating, constipation, diarrhea, and upset stomach. Although IBS can occur at any age, it usually begins in adolescence or early adulthood.

Symptoms

One of the difficulties in diagnosing and treating IBS is that its symptoms are numerous and vary from person to person. The medical profession is more comfortable with conditions that present a consistent set of symptoms.

Some of the symptoms that have been associated with IBS include diarrhea, constipation, abdominal pain and distention, colicky pain relieved by a bowel movement, bloating, intestinal gas or flatulence, bowel incontinence, excess mucus production in the colon, nausea, fatigue, anorexia, and depression.

Despite the variability in symptoms, if you have IBS, you more than likely experience abdominal pain or discomfort that is:

> **Excessive gas, diarrhea, and constipation are all major symptoms of IBS.**
>
> These symptoms…and the natural steps you can take to relieve them…are covered in more detail in Part III of this book.

- relieved with defecation,
- associated with a change in frequency of stool, or
- associated with a change in the form or appearance of the stool.

You also are likely to have:

- abnormal stool formation—either hard and lumpy or loose and watery,
- abnormal stool frequency—either more than three bowel movements a day or fewer than three a week, and
- abnormal stool passage—straining, extreme urgency, or the feeling of not being able to completely evacuate.

You can experience these stool issues intermittently, and may have mostly constipation, mostly diarrhea, or a combination of the two.

Physicians arrive at a diagnosis of IBS by the process of elimination. In other words, they rule out problems like colon cancer, intestinal blockage, structural defects in the bowel, bacterial infections, lactose intolerance, diverticulitis, laxative abuse, pancreatitis, and thyroid problems. If none of these problems can be identified, IBS often becomes the default diagnosis.

The conventional treatment for IBS has been any medication that gives symptomatic relief. Drugs are prescribed to slow the motility of the bowel (in cases of diarrhea) or increase the frequency of the stools (in cases of constipation). Antispasmodics are given for gastrointestinal cramps. Some doctors prescribe antidepressants—not necessarily to address the depression that can come with IBS, but for pain relief. And others give their patients antibiotics, thinking an overgrowth of bacteria in the small intestine may be contributing to IBS pain. (While the bacterial problem may be real, antibiotics are not the answer, as I explained earlier. Balancing your bacterial flora with probiotics is a much more effective solution.)

Ironically, many medications given to address one IBS symptom can make other symptoms worse. For instance, both antispasmodics and antidepressants can worsen constipation. And as is almost always true, these medicines offer only temporary relief of symptoms rather than a real solution to the underlying problem.

Contributing factors

Since IBS has no physical or disease basis—like inflammatory bowel disease (IBD), colon cancer, and other digestive diseases have—it's important to look for likely contributing factors to the syndrome. Also, because IBS has no organic basis, it's generally not thought to be a condition that leads to more serious diseases. Yet, this is cold comfort to those suffering through the many debilitating symptoms of IBS.

Antibiotic use

For many people, IBS first shows up after an infection—and often one in the gastrointestinal tract—particularly when a long course of potent antibiotics have been used to address the infection. Antibiotics disrupt the normal bacterial flora in the gut, and this imbalance can lead to IBS.

Food intolerance and triggers

Intolerance to certain foods is one of the primary triggers of IBS. Research shows that certain dietary items can cause the bowels to slow, resulting in constipation. Common offenders for this are dairy products, chocolate, and alcohol. And on the other side of the spectrum, diarrhea can result from intolerance to foods like lactose, fructose, or sorbitol, which is a common artificial sweetener.

In fact, one recent study suggests that fructose alone may be responsible for 30 to 60 percent of all cases of IBS. Dr. Young Choi, at the University of Iowa Carver College of Medicine, tested the effects of fructose ingestion on 183 individuals over a two-year period. He consistently found that each of the symptoms associated with IBS could be triggered with increased ingestion of fructose, and that symptoms could be eliminated by avoiding fructose intake.[19]

Caffeine, bran and wheat flour, and dietary fat can all intensify symptoms of IBS because they are GI stimulants or irritants, and can kick-start the muscles in your colon, leading to pain, bloating, diarrhea, constipation, or a combination of the two. A diet lacking in sufficient dietary fiber can exacerbate your IBS symptoms as well.

Poor digestive capability

A decrease in digestive juices and enzymes results in the incomplete breakdown of various foods. Undigested proteins, fats, and carbohydrates can all create havoc in the intestinal tract.

Protein fractions can be absorbed into the bloodstream from the small intestine and cause reactions that mimic allergies, locally as well as throughout the body. Undigested fats can ferment in warm cavities of the lower bowel and create gas or flatulence, resulting in bloating, distension, and pain. And, undigested carbohydrates can pass to the lower bowel and provide the ideal food for the growth and replication of pathogenic and disease-causing bacteria, fungi, and yeast.

As we age, our bodies are less able to produce hydrochloric acid in the stomach, which reduces our ability to break down proteins. Sluggish bile and gallbladder problems also prevent many people from properly breaking down fats in the diet. And surgical removal of the gallbladder without supplementing with bile salts probably increases the difficulty a hundredfold or more.

Stress

Earlier in this book, I discussed stress and its intimate connection with your digestive health. This seems to be particularly true with IBS. Some studies have shown that people with IBS have significantly higher stress levels than those without the condition.

Research indicates that 60% of those with IBS also suffer with a psychiatric disorder, most commonly anxiety and depression. Some theorize that people with IBS may be more sensitive to emotional problems and more sensitized to physical discomfort in the colon.

Also, it's important to note that the stress-IBS relationship runs both ways. IBS can cause stress just as surely as stress can cause IBS. Fortunately, stress reduction techniques have been shown to help relieve symptoms for some suffering with IBS and can short-circuit this debilitating cycle.

Other factors

In addition to these main categories of IBS contributing factors, there are others including: genetics, drugs, radiation therapy, smoking, alcohol use or abuse, carbonated beverages, lack of sleep and exercise, surgical trauma or injury to the bowel, eating disorders, and use of hormones—particularly oral contraceptives or hormone replacement therapy.

⁍ Your Action Plan for IBS ⁍

I've found that successful treatment of IBS requires a multi-faceted approach.

1. **Eat a healthy, low-fat, high-fiber diet.** As with any digestive condition, a healthy diet is critical for recovery. Start with the diet basics I've already outlined in this book. But be aware of these specific points.

   - First, because many people with IBS have sensitivities to wheat and bran, these are generally not the best sources of fiber for your diet. Instead, focus on water-soluble fibers that promote the formation of protective gel and mucus in the bowel. This type of fiber is found in guar gum, psyllium or Indian husks, oat bran, flax seeds, fruits, vegetables and legumes. An excellent source for psyllium husks and guar gum, as well as yeast and additive-free vitamins, is Freeda Vitamins (*freedavitamins.com* or 1-800-777-3737).

   - Keep in mind that when you increase the fiber in your diet, you must also increase the amount of water you drink. This is because fiber absorbs and binds with water, creating the extra bulk necessary to gently stimulate and "sweep clean" your colon.

   - Also, although increasing your intake of fruits and vegetables is important for treating IBS, during periods of diarrhea they should be avoided and then slowly reintroduced when your bowels return to normal.

   - Eliminate sugar and highly concentrated sugar-containing products like fruit juices from your diet. Avoid alcoholic beverages. And stay away from tomatoes and tomato products, which can irritate your sensitive bowel.

   - Minimize your consumption of salt water fish and those from lakes contaminated from acid rain. This caution also applies to canned tuna. Although most individuals will experience no such problems, German research has found that the mercury often contained in these fish is one of the main triggers for IBS episodes.

   - If you have severe IBS, you may need to go on an elimination-type diet for two weeks or so. By restricting the diet to chicken, lamb, potatoes, rice and fruits, and then gradually adding other foods one at a time, you can often determine which food triggers are contributing to your symptoms and avoid these in the future.

     To make it easier to identify which foods are your triggers, keep a daily log of what you eat and the symptoms you're experiencing.

2. **Reestablish a healthy bacterial balance in your colon.** As I've said many times, this is an essential step for good digestive health and overall wellness,

but it's especially critical if you suffer from IBS. Eating lactic acid–fermented foods, like homemade sauerkraut is one the best ways to do this. You can also eat live-culture yogurt and take daily probiotic supplements. I would venture to say that incorporating probiotics into the daily diet could eliminate 75 to 80 percent of all IBS cases.

3. **Speed your body's return to gut health with hydrogen peroxide.** To help eliminate any infectious pathogens that might be present in your gut you can use hydrogen peroxide drops to introduce oxygen into your bowels. Pathogenic bacteria, cancer cells, and most of the other harmful "bugs" are anaerobic, meaning they survive only in environments without oxygen. On the other hand, beneficial bacteria need and love oxygen. That's why they're called aerobic bacteria.

Use 1–2 drops of 3 percent hydrogen peroxide, taken three times a day on an empty stomach. I recommend starting with 35 percent food grade hydrogen peroxide and diluting it down to three percent with distilled water, rather than using the three percent hydrogen peroxide being sold over the counter. This means mixing approximately 11 parts distilled water with 1 part food grade hydrogen peroxide.

If you're unable, or don't care to mix your own hydrogen peroxide, there are several products on the market that will probably accomplish the same effect. The only kicker is that you'll pay a lot more for the convenience. One such product is called Aerobic 07 from Aerobic Life (*aerobiclife.com* or 1-800-798-0707). The recommended dosage for this product is 20 drops in a glass of water taken three times daily on an empty stomach.

4. **Soothe your irritated bowels with slippery elm.** Slippery elm powder is a favorite topical remedy of Native Americans for wounds, burns, and boils. And it's also used internally to soothe an irritated intestinal system.

You can purchase slippery elm in bulk or in capsules (I prefer the bulk product) in most health food stores or from companies such as Penn Herb (*PennHerb.com* or 1-800-523-9971), or from Kalyx.com (*Kalyx.com* or 1-315-245-3000).

A slippery elm drink can be made by adding a heaping teaspoon of the powder to a little cold water to make a paste, and then pouring on a cup of boiling water while constantly stirring the mixture. Let it cool and then drink it, three times a day. For a slight variation you can use boiling milk instead of water and flavor the mixture with cinnamon or nutmeg. If you take slippery elm as a supplement, I suggest 2 capsules (400 or 500 mg each) three or four times daily.

5. **Or try another soothing agent called Sialex.** An alternative to slippery elm is a product called Sialex from Ecological Formulas. It contains an extract of mucin, the main component of mucus, that re-establishes the protective mucus layer in the bowel and provides a lubricating action.

You shouldn't need Sialex if you use slippery elm, but I wanted you to know about it because it's helpful in healing the most stubborn cases of IBS. The recommended dosage is 1 to 3 capsules with meals. It can be purchased on the Web from *Netriceuticals.com* or 1-888-852-4993.

6. **Add aloe vera to the mix.** If your colon is extremely irritated, ¼ cup of aloe vera gel (not liquid) daily between meals will speed the healing process. If the taste is objectionable, mix the gel with non–sugar added fruit juice. This gel is available in local health food and grocery stores.

7. **Consider peppermint to ease bowel pain.** Peppermint has long been revered as an effective remedy for gastrointestinal distress and it has several very helpful healing characteristics.

It has a gentle disinfecting effect that helps prevent the fermentation of improperly digested foods in the stomach and bowels. This helps prevent the formation of intestinal gas and the pain associated with it. It also promotes normal liver and gallbladder function, which are crucial to proper digestion. And it's a well-known antispasmodic. It relaxes the muscles of the intestinal tract and prevents colon spasms typical of IBS.

Peppermint tea bags are readily available in both supermarkets and health food stores. The tea can also be made from fresh leaves. Simply add 1 or 2 teaspoons to a cup of hot, not boiling, water and let it stand covered for 10 to 15 minutes. I would recommend keeping a supply of peppermint tea around the house. However, don't use it on a casual, regular basis. Use it only during periods of stomach upset. Regular habitual use will lessen its effect.

Since the active menthol ingredients in peppermint are rapidly absorbed in the stomach and upper GI tract, taking peppermint in the form of tea will have little, if any, effect on the lower bowels. With IBS, you want to deliver the healing constituents to your colon, too.

For this, you'll need to take enteric-coated peppermint oil capsules. European studies have found that these enteric-coated capsules are very effective in treating IBS.[20]

These capsules are available in the United States under the name Mentharil by PhytoPharmica (*phytostore.com* or 1-877-241-8822). The dosage generally recommended for IBS patients is 2–3 capsules a day taken between meals. The only side effect noted has been a temporary burning sensation in the rectal area after a bowel movement. This comes from excess, unabsorbed menthol. It poses no danger and can be alleviated by simply reducing the dosage.

8. **Try therapeutic heat.** Applying topical heat directly to your gut can be a simple and surprisingly effective way to relieve the pain of colon spasms commonly associated with IBS. Intense heat relaxes the colon, bringing soothing relief without side effects. A heating pad, hot water bottle, or hot pack applied directly to your abdomen is most effective.

Heat can also be used proactively to head off IBS attacks triggered by stress. Regular jacuzzi, steam bath or sauna sessions can do wonders mentally and physically.

9. **Reduce your stress.** Because stress can trigger IBS symptoms or make existing symptoms worse, it's important to effectively manage your daily stress. As I mentioned earlier, you need to find the stress relief techniques that work best for your personality and lifestyle. Deep breathing, exercise, prayer and spirituality, laughter, music, meditation, and holistic health practices are all methods to consider.

Behavioral therapy has also been shown to help relieve stress and stress-related symptoms for those suffering with IBS. This can include biofeedback, hypnosis, cognitive behavior therapy, and traditional psychotherapy.

The Diet of Last Resort

It's rare not to see significant improvement or resolution of bowel problems with the steps listed in Your Action Plan for IBS. But, if your case is particularly severe or entrenched, you may need something more rigorous when it comes to dietary changes.

There is a program called "the Specific Carbohydrate Diet," developed by Dr. Sidney Haas and described in his book, *Management of Celiac Disease*, which I have found very helpful for such cases. It takes a lot of discipline and a continuing commitment, but it will work.

His groundbreaking research and dietary developments were later refined by Elaine Gottschall, who used her education in nutritional biochemistry and cellular biology, as well as her personal experience with a daughter suffering with chronic ulcerative colitis, to write her own book, *Breaking the Vicious Cycle*—now in its 11th printing. Gottschall's book explains the program in detail, presents the scientific rationale, and outlines which foods are "legal" and which are "illegal" in the diet. Her program involves some significant changes in the way most people eat but it has been a godsend to thousands.

Some of Gottschall's recommendations conflict with what I've suggested for IBS. For example, she felt slippery elm and other mucilaginous herbs contain starches that feed pathogens in the bowels. Most of what I've recommended, however, doesn't conflict with her program. As I said before, if the regimen and program I first outlined doesn't work for you, then I highly recommend following the Specific Carbohydrate Diet.

See "Diet Therapy" on pages 67-68 in the Inflammatory Bowel Disease section of this book for more details on the diet and where to get your own copy of Gottschall's informative book.

Food Allergies

A food allergy is an immune system reaction that takes place in your body after you eat a certain food. These allergies affect an estimated 11 to 15 million Americans and have been on the rise in recent years.

A primary reason for this is what I call the "sad SAD diet," meaning the sorry Standard American Diet. An average American diet is loaded with sugar, processed oils, and other refined ingredients. Additionally, many food products on the market today contain chemicals such as sulfites, food stabilizers, and artificial colorings and flavorings, which can aggravate allergies. Some researchers believe that high amounts of chemical pollutants and contaminants, such as pesticides and herbicides, also have increased our susceptibility to food allergies.

Another contributing factor to food allergies that doesn't get much attention is emotional stress. It appears that people are more prone to food allergies when they are experiencing extremely stressful situations in their lives. The exact connection is not yet clear, but the negative impact stress puts on the immune system is a likely factor.

Immediate vs. delayed food allergies

Some food allergies are obvious because they have extreme symptoms that show up within minutes of eating the trigger food. An example is when a child starts wheezing right after eating a peanut. These are called immediate allergies.

Decades ago, researchers found that patients with immediate allergies had elevated levels of an antibody called immunoglobulin E (IgE) during their allergy attacks. But, they incorrectly concluded that, if you don't have elevated IgE, you don't have a food allergy—just a food sensitivity or intolerance.

We now know that there's more than one way the immune system can respond to a food allergy. Non-IgE, or delayed, allergies—which are just as common as immediate allergies—appear hours or even days after eating a particular food. Delayed allergies involve different components of the immune system, but they cause the same wide variety of symptoms.

Common triggers

While any food can cause an allergic reaction, proteins seem to be more allergenic than fats and carbohydrates. Some of the more common food allergy reactions are triggered by a tough kind of food protein that resists the heat and digestive juices that break down other proteins.

Most food allergies are triggered by proteins in: peanuts and tree nuts, like walnuts and pecans; shellfish, such as shrimp, lobster, and crab; eggs, and milk. Other common food allergens are seeds, soybeans, coconut, celery, carrots, members of the nightshade family (tomatoes, white potatoes, bell peppers, hot peppers, and eggplant), and gluten (especially wheat).

Although these are the most common food allergy triggers, people can also have an allergic response to food additives and to foods that do not have a high protein content at all.

Nature and nurture

You can be born with food allergies, but you also can develop them during your life if you get sensitized to a certain food or ingredient. This happens when your body mistakenly identifies a particular food substance as something harmful and triggers your immune system to release IgE antibodies. With subsequent exposure to the same food substance, the IgE antibodies remember the offending substance and signal your immune system to release histamines and other chemicals to "protect" your body.

Because repeated exposure is part of the food allergy process, it makes sense that certain foods are more common allergy triggers in some cultures than in others. For instance, allergies to fish are especially common in Scandinavia, and the same goes for allergies to rice in Asia, peanuts in the U.S., celery in Europe, buckwheat in South Korea, and peaches in Mediterranean countries.[21]

It's also interesting to note that you're at increased risk of having food allergies if other allergies, asthma, eczema, or hives run in your family. You can outgrow food allergies, but they can also come back later in life. Childhood food allergies that are usually outgrown include those to milk, soy, wheat, and eggs. On the other hand, severe childhood allergies and allergies to nuts and shellfish tend to be lifelong conditions.

? **Did You Know…**

If you're allergic to one food, you're at increased risk for becoming allergic to others. In fact, certain food allergies tend to run together. Also, if you're allergic to something other than food—like pollen or mold—you also are at increased risk for developing a food allergy.

Weakened natural defenses

Other factors that contribute to your risk of developing food allergies have to do with your overall wellness and the strength of your natural digestive system. If your body lacks important nutrients or if you suffer from chronic inflammation and stress, the integrity of your intestinal lining may be compromised and less effective at keeping allergens from being absorbed.

Another important factor is your body's ability to produce strong stomach acids to break down stubborn allergenic proteins before they can travel to your intestines where they can be absorbed. This acid production ability commonly diminishes with age.

Your body must also balance its potent stomach acid with a strong buffering system so that you can maintain a slightly alkaline pH in your blood and body tissue. Without this balance, enzymes that break down proteins into smaller amino acid components can get destroyed. As a result, incomplete protein molecules can be absorbed into your bloodstream and circulate throughout your body. These proteins are notorious for causing all types of allergic reactions, in particular those related to breathing and skin irritation.

Be Prepared If Your Food Allergy Is Severe

If your food allergy is severe, you need to have a game plan in place to take immediate action in the event of an anaphylactic reaction.

You should carry a self-injector of epinephrine with you at all times or, for children, give the injector to a supervising adult and make sure he or she knows how to use it. If you use epinephrine, you should go to the emergency room immediately so your condition can be monitored.

You should also always wear a medical alert bracelet to let emergency medical personnel know of your condition, so they can react quickly with the correct treatment.

The number one cause of anaphylaxis-related death is the delayed use of epinephrine. So don't delay. Make sure you're prepared in the event of an allergy emergency.

Food allergy reactions

Food allergy reactions can vary according to the person and the severity of the allergy, but common reactions include digestive symptoms, like abdominal pain, diarrhea, nausea or vomiting; hives, itching, or eczema; wheezing, nasal congestion, or trouble breathing; swelling of the tongue, throat, lips, face, or other parts of the body; and dizziness, lightheadedness, or fainting.

If you have a severe food allergy, it can cause anaphylaxis, which is a serious allergic reaction with widespread effects on the body. Symptoms include: constriction of your airways; swollen throat that makes it difficult to breathe; rapid pulse; dizziness and lightheadedness; shock, with a severe drop in blood pressure; loss of consciousness; and even death.

The first sign of an anaphylactic reaction, however, often shows up on your skin in the form of a rash, hives, itching, or redness. Some people also experience a feeling of extreme anxiety—most likely because their body is going into chemical overdrive.

Diagnosing a food allergy

Diagnosing immediate food allergies is as simple as getting a blood test to check for elevated IgE levels. But a delayed food allergy is more elusive to diagnose. The best way takes some time and effort on your part, and involves a bit of detective work. Here's how:

First, record the details of your eating and digestive symptoms. For at least two weeks, list every single item you eat or drink. Write down how much you eat and when, how the food was prepared, and how you feel throughout the day and even the next day. If you eat any packaged foods, list the ingredients. If you experience any discomfort, include a note about when symptoms started and how long they lasted. You should list your medications and supplements, too, so you can have a complete picture of your nutrient and chemical intake.

Next, practice an elimination diet. Start removing common foods from your diet—one at a time—for two to six weeks per food item. Note any improvement in your symptoms and make a note of which food eliminations preceded the improvements. If your food allergies are severe, once you've identified your personal food triggers, avoid them permanently.

If your food allergies are mild to moderate, you can move on to the next step, which is reintroducing foods to retest and confirm your food triggers and to re-evaluate your body's immune system response to them.

Here, you add each of your trigger foods back into your diet, one food per day. Eat the suspect food as part of at least two meals that day, making sure you don't introduce other potential allergens at the same time. Record the date and time you reintroduced each food, and note any immediate and delayed reactions that you experience.

If you experience a reaction to a particular food, stop eating it and take note of it so you can be sure to eliminate it from your diet permanently. Before you reintroduce any new food, make sure that you have been symptom-free for at least two days. Repeat this testing with all your suspected trigger foods until you figure out exactly which ones incite an immune system reaction.

Knowing which foods are your personal allergy triggers is a huge step toward freedom from the pain and suffering brought on by food allergies. But, there is more you can do. These are outlined below.

▮▮▶ Your Action Plan for Food Allergies ▮▮▶

1. **Avoid the foods that you've determined are your allergy triggers.** An allergic response is also an inflammatory response, and every time inflammation occurs, it weakens your immune system and increases your allergic tendencies.

2. **Rotate the foods that you are able to eat** so that you don't consume any particular item more than once every four days. Include beverages, condiments, and oils in this rotation strategy. Preventing overexposure to foods in this way will reduce your sensitivity to them and also reduce your chances of developing allergies.

3. **Incorporate bone broth into your diet.** In Part I of this book, I mentioned the many benefits of adding bone broth to your diet, and one of these was that it appears to help protect against food allergies. This is because bone broth is rich in the amino acid glycine, which helps promote gastrointestinal mucosal integrity and function. Food allergies are often the result of undigested food particles making their way into the bloodstream, where they're treated as foreign. Glycine helps increase the production of hydrochloric acid in the stomach, and food gets digested more completely in the higher-acid environment. See page 15 for details on making your own healthy bone broth.

4. **Consider a gentle detoxification program** to cleanse accumulated toxins from your body. This will make it easier for your liver to manage your day-to-day toxin load and also improve the strength of your intestinal mucosa barrier, which can help prevent the absorption of allergens into your body. Go to pages 138–139 for more details on the detoxification steps I recommend.

5. **To help strengthen your body's ability to tolerate allergenic foods** without over-reacting to them, take these dietary supplements:

   - A high-potency daily **multi-nutrient**

   - **Bioflavonoids**, 500–1,000 mg twice a day

   - **Mineral-buffered vitamin C**, 2,000–5,000 mg a day in divided doses. (Cut back if you experience stomach upset or diarrhea.)

   - **Pantothenic acid**, 250–500 mg twice a day

   - **Flaxseed oil**, 1–2 tablespoons per day

- **Digestive enzymes**, 500 mg of bromelain two to four times a day and 200–300 mg of papain two to four times a day. To enhance digestion, take these enzymes with food. To help decrease inflammation, take them between meals.

6. **If you eat a trigger food by mistake, try this stop-gap remedy.** While it's best to completely avoid your food triggers, it's not always possible. If your food allergy reactions are generally mild-to-medium, consider using this quick, easy measure to soothe symptoms when you inadvertently eat a trigger food.

   Simply take a dose of Alka-Seltzer Gold (antacid formula) or Alka-Aid (available in health food stores). Both of these products are alkali compounds and can help fortify your stomach acid buffering system, which should minimize absorption of allergens into your bloodstream. If you take one at the first sign of symptoms, you should start to see an improvement within 10 or 15 minutes. Be sure to note the offending foods for future reference and to only use this step as a "once-in–a-great-while" stop-gap measure!

•*Track Your Success!*• • • • • • • • • • • • • • • • • • • •

To track your success with this Action Plan, I highly recommend that you record the exact steps you're taking to address your food allergies each day, as well as the symptoms you are experiencing at the time, and how you are feeling emotionally.

Putting these details on paper is an excellent way to see what works for you. It's also a great way to document the improvements you're experiencing and just how far you've come using safe, natural solutions to your digestive problem.

Turn to pages 135–136 for sample pages that makes tracking this information simple. Use these pages as your master copy and photocopy more pages to fill in with your details.

Inflammatory Bowel Disease

Inflammatory bowel disease (IBD) consists of two different, chronic diseases that cause inflammation of the intestines—ulcerative colitis (UC) and Crohn's disease (CD). It's estimated that more than 1 million Americans suffer with these serious diseases and they account for 700,000 physician visits and 100,000 hospitalizations per year.[22]

IBD typically affects people ages 15 to 30, but it can afflict those younger and older. And it seems to afflict people in North American and Europe more than anywhere else in the world, suggesting a genetic component to the disease. Approximately 10 to 20 percent of people with IBD have one or more family members affected with it as well.[23]

The "D" makes a difference

Although the acronyms sound similar and they share some symptoms, IBD is not like IBS. As discussed earlier, IBS is a "functional" disorder, where the digestive system looks normal, but doesn't work as expected. It is not a disease, but rather a syndrome with a defined group of symptoms, most commonly abdominal pain or discomfort, along with diarrhea, constipation, or alternating bouts of the two.

On the other hand, UC and CD are autoimmune diseases that lead to chronic inflammation and subsequent damage to the GI tract lining and beyond. For this reason, IBD is considered more serious than IBS. It can cause permanent harm to the intestines

---

Celiac Disease

Like UC and CD, celiac disease is an autoimmune disease of the intestine, but it's not considered an inflammatory bowel disease. This chronic digestive condition, which is sometimes referred to as celiac sprue or gluten sensitive enteropathy (GSE), is triggered by eating gluten, a protein found in bread, pasta, cookies, and many other foods containing wheat, barley, rye, and possibly oats. Signs and symptoms of celiac disease include diarrhea, constipation, abdominal pain, gas, bloating, lactose intolerance, nausea, vomiting, decreased appetite, unexplained weight loss, and stools that float.

With celiac disease, the small projections—called villi—that line the small intestine and absorb nutrients become flattened by immune system attack and are unable to function properly. This can dramatically affect nutrient absorption, with obvious impact throughout your body. In fact, long-term symptoms of celiac disease include anemia, bone and joint pain, osteoporosis, depression, fatigue, growth delay in children, hair loss, hypoglycemia, malnutrition, skin disorders, and vitamin deficiencies, to name a few.

Blood tests can be performed to detect specific antibodies associated with the disease. And if celiac disease is suspected, an endoscopy is usually performed to confirm. The treatment is dietary and involves removing all damaging grains from the foods you eat. This one lifestyle change has the power to completely reverse the progress of celiac disease, allowing you to return to a healthy, symptom-free life.

---

and intestinal bleeding, as well as complications that can require surgery and treatment with powerful steroids and immunosuppressant drugs.

Also, the risk of colon cancer in UC patients increases significantly above that of the general population about 8 to 10 years after diagnosis. And the risk is greatest in those whose whole colon is affected by the disease. The risk of colon cancer for CD patients is similar to UC patients, plus there is an increased risk of cancer in the small intestine as well. Some studies suggest that people with IBD are five times more likely to develop colon cancer than the general public, and that this risk is consistent regardless of whether symptoms have been active or in remission.[24]

As with other autoimmune diseases, UC and CD are a result of the immune system misinterpreting signals in the body and "attacking" parts of itself—in this case, the digestive tract. Medical experts now believe that a genetic defect may be responsible for these abnormal signals and immune response. But, environment and lifestyle factors also play a role, and are likely the catalysts that initiate the onset and flare-ups of the disease. Both UC and CD tend to alternate between periods of remission and relapses with active symptoms.

Stress as a trigger

There have been numerous theories as to which, if any, outside factors contribute to IBD flare-ups, including smoking, NSAID or antibiotic use, and infections such as colds and pneumonia. But the one factor that has gotten the most attention recently is stress.

While the precise connection between stress and IBD flare-ups is unclear, researchers believe that the sympathetic nervous system, which kicks into gear when you're under stress, affects the lining of the colon and might aggravate any existing inflammation. They also suggest that stress hormones may help create a hospitable environment in the bowels for bad bacteria, thereby upsetting your balance of bacterial flora and setting the stage for IBD symptoms to return or worsen.

A new study conducted by Canadian researchers and published in the *American Journal of Gastroenterology*, found that among bowel-disease patients they followed for a year, the risk of a symptom flare-up increased when patients were feeling particularly stressed.

Specifically, 552 men and women with UC or CD were asked to complete surveys every three months for one year. The surveys asked about symptom flare-ups, stressful events, and perceived stress—which was defined as how well they felt they could deal with their daily stresses.

The researchers found that a patient's risk of a symptom flare-up increased by more than twofold when they had reported high levels of perceived stress in the preceding three-month period. And of patients who reported a flare-up, 52 percent had had high perceived stress levels in the preceding three months, compared with 29 percent of those who remained symptom free.[25]

Previous research has indicated that people with IBD feel that stress worsens their symptoms, but this study is one of the first to show scientific evidence that the perception of stress has a direct and significant impact on the course of the disease.

Ulcerative colitis

UC primarily affects the rectum and areas of the colon near the rectum. But, it can spread to the entire colon in some people. With UC, the inner mucosal lining of the intestines becomes inflamed and develops ulcers. It causes abdominal pain, gas, and frequent diarrhea, along with feces tinged with blood and mucus. Sometimes, if the rectum becomes severely inflamed—a condition known as proctitis—it can lead to constipation as well.

Crohn's disease

CD, unlike UC, most commonly attacks the end section of your small intestine, also referred to as your terminal ileum. Less often, it affects the large intestine and other parts of the digestive tract as well. While UC creates ulcerative sores in the mucosal lining of

PART II

Don't Overlook Toothpaste & Dish Detergents

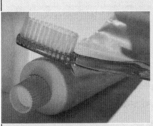

There are two surprising contributors to bowel inflammation that have been constantly overlooked, but I want you to be aware of them—toothpaste and dish detergent.

Toothpaste can be an irritant to the gastrointestinal tract when swallowed, particularly the newer toothpastes that contain even more potent antibacterial compounds. While most of us avoid swallowing toothpaste, it can be a problem in the very young or the elderly. This is definitely something that should be considered in anyone who suffers from Crohn's disease, ulcerative colitis, IBS, or other bowel problems.

I have yet to read about the link that likely exists between dish detergents and bowel inflammation. Detergent residue can be extremely irritating to the intestinal tract. Every year, there are more and more advertisements promoting the stronger grease-cutting abilities of dish detergents. Manufacturers of detergents do test the toxicity of their products on rats, but not on humans. I can't help but suspect that individuals with chronic bowel inflammation are sensitive to these residues.

If you suffer with a bowel inflammatory condition, take extra care to thoroughly rinse all dishes and eating utensils. Mothers with infants also need to be careful. I would suspect that many cases of infant diarrhea are directly linked to detergent residue.

In the 1980s, one study estimated that adults ingest anywhere from 0.3 to 75 milligrams a day of detergent residue, while bottle-fed infants are taking in closer to 250 milligrams. The problem is obviously more prevalent with hand-washing than with automatic dishwashers, most of which have a long rinse cycle. In either case, use the minimum amount of detergent necessary for the job, and rinse very well.

---

the gut, CD attacks much deeper, with damage extending to other layers of the intestinal wall. CD can also result in anal skin tags, abscesses, and fistulas, or abnormal connections between loops of the intestine.

Symptoms of CD are much like those of UC, starting with abdominal pain, gas, and diarrhea. Constipation can become a problem as well with CD if inflammation and damage to the intestinal wall is great enough to create a partial obstruction—called a stricture.

Other shared symptoms and complications

Diarrhea is a major symptom in both UC and CD, and it can lead to complications such as dehydration, a rapid heartbeat, and low blood pressure. The loss of fluids caused by diarrhea can also lead to nutrient loss, malnutrition, weight loss, fever, fatigue, and further abdominal pain as the nerves and muscles of the intestines become irritated.

Furthermore, the chronic inflammation associated with UC and CD can lead to a host of other complications that reach beyond the digestive tract. Research has shown that those with IBD tend to have inflammation throughout the body, affecting the heart, skin, liver, eyes, mouth, and joints. Anemia due to blood loss is also a shared symptom. And the nutrient loss associated with IBD has been linked to growth problems and delayed puberty in children and teens with the condition.

? **Did You Know...**

There is a clear, but not well-publicized connection between colon ailments and cardiovascular disease.

Before World War I, 57 leading British physicians gathered at the Royal Society of Medicine in London to discuss how inflammation and toxicity from the colon can affect many organs, including the heart.

They called it "alimentary toxemia," and concluded that degeneration and weakening of the heart muscle, fatty degeneration of the heart, low blood pressure, high blood pressure, enlargement of the heart, dilation of the aorta, and arteriosclerosis were all causatively associated with digestive tract disorder.[26]

Subsequent research supports the connection. For instance, in a 2007 study that appeared in the *Journal of the American Medical Association*, researchers in Hong Kong found a significant incidence of colorectal tumors—50 percent—among patients diagnosed with major coronary artery disease. Researchers cited inflammation as a potential reason these conditions co-occur, similar to the dynamic with smoking and insulin resistance. [27]

Making a diagnosis

Diagnosing IBD is not simple. For one thing, both UC and CD can progress for years without obvious symptoms. And once symptoms do appear, they can be confused with numerous other digestive conditions, including IBS.

Screening for IBD usually involves bloods tests to check for signs of inflammation in the body and examination of stool samples to see if there is any blood present. More invasive testing includes a sigmoidoscopy or colonoscopy, where a long, thin tube with a tiny camera attached is inserted through the anus so the doctor can take a look at the intestinal walls and determine if there is inflammation, bleeding, or ulcers, and can take a small sample, or biopsy, of the intestinal wall for further laboratory analysis.

A sigmoidoscopy only extends through the rectum and lower end of the colon, while a colonoscopy is an examination of the full length of the colon. (For more details concerning colonoscopy and how to best prepare for the procedure, see pages 82–84.)

Similarly, your doctor may want to do an upper endoscopy, which is similar to a colonoscopy, but the tube is directed down the throat and into the esophagus, stomach, and duodenum.

Your doctor can use other technology to take a "look" at your GI tract without actually inserting equipment inside your body. One way is with a barium study. For this test, you must first drink a barium solution, which allows your intestines to be seen on X-ray film. X-rays are then taken, and the doctor uses these to evaluate the condition of your GI tract.

A computerized tomography (CT) scan is a similar, but even more precise, X-ray. For this, you are required to ingest or get an IV infusion of a contrast dye. Your doctor can also make use of ultrasound, which involves sound waves to create a "picture" of your pelvic organs. It is usually used to detect gallstones and abscesses, which are complications of CD. Finally, there is magnetic resonance imaging (MRI) technology, which uses radio waves and superconducting magnets to create images of your internal organs. This technology is generally used to detect fistulas and abscesses that are complications of CD.

Traditional treatment

Once a diagnosis of IBD is made, doctors traditionally prescribe anti-inflammatory drugs, such as aminosalicylates (Azulfidine, Asacol, Pentasa, Colazal) and the more powerful corticosteroids, like prednisone (Deltasone), methylprednisolone (Medrol), and hydrocortisone, to bring the active disease under control and into remission. Then immunosuppressants or immunomodulators, like azathioprine (Imuran, Azasan) and 6-mercaptopurine (6-MP, Purinethol) are added to try to keep the disease in remission.

Although the fast-acting corticosteroids are valuable for quickly addressing severe inflammation, they have a long, long list of undesirable side effects, from weight gain, acne, and mood swings to high blood pressure, psychosis, cataracts, insomnia, and osteoporosis.

And the immune-modulating medications also have a laundry list of side effects, too, including many of the symptoms you are already trying to avoid, such as diarrhea, nausea, and malaise. They can also contribute to inflammation of the pancreas and bone marrow suppression, which can lead to increased risk of infection or serious bleeding.

Surgery is often performed to address the IBD damage done to the intestines. For UC, surgery is considered when a person can't tolerate or doesn't respond to medication or if there are precancerous or cancerous changes in the colon. For many years, surgery meant removal of the colon, requiring the patient to have a permanent soma, or external bag used to drain stool. But more recently, surgeons instead create a reservoir out of the lower part of the small intestine and connect it to the anus for more normal defecation.

For CD, surgery is often performed when a patient doesn't respond to medications or has complications of the disease, such as abscesses, strictures, or fistulas. In these surgeries, only the affected part of the colon is removed. Unfortunately, surgery is a common course of traditional treatment for CD. In fact, it's estimated that 70 percent of those with CD undergo surgery for their disease. And even this drastic measure isn't enough to keep CD at bay. Statistics show that the risk of the disease returning within 10 to 15 years after surgery is approximately 70 to 85 percent.[28]

Diet therapy

If powerful medicines with devastating side effects and surgeries with life-altering outcomes and questionable success aren't the path you want to take, there are other options for you to try. (As is always the case with serious medical conditions, make your treatment choices and carry them out under the supervision of your doctor.)

One powerful, all-natural "therapy" for IBD is the Specific Carbohydrate Diet. As I mentioned in the IBS section of this book, this diet has proven to be nothing short of a miracle for thousands upon thousands of people suffering with serious bowel disorders.

The late Elaine Gottschall, promulgator of the diet, learned firsthand about the devastating effects of bowel disease in 1955, when her four-year-old daughter was diagnosed with "incurable" ulcerative colitis. Specialists recommended a colectomy. Resolved to spare her child the operation, Gottschall discovered a 92-year-old physician, Dr. Sidney Haas, who had devised the diet.

After two years on the diet, her daughter was free of symptoms, and after another few years, was able to eat a normal diet. Determined to understand why the diet worked, Gottschall, at age 47, plunged into science courses after studying the effects of various sugars on the digestive tract and eventually attained a master of science from the University of Western Ontario.

She wrote several books to share her wealth of knowledge and experience with others who are searching for natural solutions to ulcerative colitis, including *Breaking the Vicious Cycle: Intestinal Health Through Diet*, available in stores, online at *Amazon.com*, or from the publisher: Kirkton Press Ltd. in Canada at 905-349-3443. Her website, *BreakingTheViciousCycle.info* is also extremely helpful. It's filled with information and links to support groups that will help you stick to the diet for the 1–2 years necessary to allow your GI tract to heal.

Cereal grains are out

The Specific Carbohydrate Diet calls for eliminating all cereal grains, including corn, oats, wheat, rye, rice, and buckwheat. This means that all bread, cake, crackers, cookies, cereals, flour, or pasta containing these grains are strictly forbidden. You'll use ground nuts in place of flour. Also out are milk and all sweeteners, except honey.

The diet consists of fresh fruits, vegetables, including legumes, as well as meat, eggs, homemade yogurt, certain cheeses, and certain nuts. You should restrict your intake of raw fruits and vegetables, though, until your diarrhea symptoms subside.

Starve intestinal microbes to vanquish your symptoms

How can eliminating grains cure diarrhea and other intestinal problems? As Gottschall explained: "When intestinal problems occur, the intestinal cells cannot produce the necessary enzymes to complete digestion of carbohydrates and, consequently, these sugars and starches remain in the intestinal tract and, upon reaching the colon, ferment." The byproducts of these unabsorbed, undigested carbohydrates—yeast and bacteria—cause diarrhea, excess gas, cramping, and distention.

By restricting carbohydrates in the diet, you "starve out" the intestinal microbes. Deprived of the food they subsist on, these harmful microbes and their byproducts eventually die out.

An astounding success rate

Based on her work as a nutritional consultant, Gottschall estimated that the diet has an 80 percent recovery rate for UC and CD and a 95 percent success rate for diverticulosis—a condition where small sac-like swellings develop in the walls of the lowest part of the colon.

If you follow the diet faithfully for three weeks, you should experience enough improvement to demonstrate the healing potential of the diet and to motivate you to continue. And Gottschall found that following the diet for a year or two can solve the underlying digestive problem, allowing you to move from the strict dietary rules of the Specific Carbohydrate Diet, to a less restrictive diet, (but one that's wholesome, nutritious, high in fiber, and low in unhealthy fat).

As I mentioned earlier, this diet isn't easy to follow and takes dedication. But, if you've lived with the pain and debilitation of IBD, it can be a true godsend. Faithful followers of the diet have formed several listserver groups to share their experiences and advice. If you're interested in joining, contact the facilitators at *rturet@optonline.com* or *SCD-list-subscribe@longisland.com*.

Following the Specific Carbohydrate Diet is a long-term commitment for ending your IBD. But there are other things you can do right away to find relief from symptoms and nurture your bowels. Just follow the Action Plan on the next page.

⏵ Your Action Plan for Inflammatory Bowel Disease ⏵

1. **Take organic, high-quality aloe vera.** This will help to accomplish a primary goal, and that is to soothe your lower bowel by decreasing inflammation there. Look for "whole" aloe vera gel, not products with aloe juice in them. You should be able to find products like this in most health food stores. I suggest taking about 2 ounces, six to eight times a day, on an empty stomach. Stick with this regimen for several weeks, even if your symptoms, like diarrhea, stop before then.

   You can make the aloe vera even more effective by adding a teaspoon of liquid chlorophyll every time you take the aloe vera. Two chlorophyll products I highly recommend are the one by Nature's Way and the one under Bernard Jenson's label. Both are readily available in most health food stores.

2. **Quickly restore good bacteria and correct the pH of your colon with lactic acid wafers.** This product, which has been produced by Standard Process Laboratories since 1939, contains a mycelium type of yeast (*Saccharomyces cerevisiae*) that converts all carbohydrates into lactic acid. I haven't found another supplement that is as effective at stopping diarrhea and helping re-establish bacterial flora of the lower bowel.

   If you're experiencing diarrhea, chew 2 lactic acid wafer tablets, three times a day with food. Continue this for at least two or three months. Once your diarrhea has stopped, you can cut back to one wafer with each meal, provided your diarrhea stays under control.

   Standard Process products aren't sold to consumers through the Internet but can be purchased by calling Village Green Apothecary at 1-800-869-9159. You can also call Standard Process' doctor referral line at 1-800-558-8740 to find a local doctor who can order the lactic acid wafers for you.

3. **Consider a 3–4 day diet limited to freshly made applesauce and white rice**, if your diarrhea is severe. It will give your intestines a chance to stabilize, while providing sufficient nutrients to prevent you from feeling lethargic.

4. **If, after following steps 1–3, you're still experiencing diarrhea, try using butyric acid enemas.** Butyric acid is naturally produced by cells in the colon through the fermentation of fiber, and is the main source of energy for the cells lining the large intestine. German studies have repeatedly shown that butyric acid enemas can reduce diarrhea, inflammation, and the discharge of blood in Crohn's disease and ulcerative colitis.

Butyric acid is generally only available through doctors. A company called Tyler Encapsulations makes a kit that contains everything you need to give butyric acid enemas for two weeks. This is the time period used in the German studies, and should be adequate to restore a balance in the colon. The kit is available from Key Pharmacy at 1-800-878-1322.

5. **Drink plenty of liquids**, especially during bouts of diarrhea. The diarrhea that comes with IBD can quickly cause you to become dehydrated, which can affect virtually every organ and system in your body.

    Water is usually a good choice, but if your diarrhea is severe, you should drink a beverage that can also restore your electrolyte balance. I like HEED sports drinks by Hammer Nutrition. They are formulated for endurance athletes and are made from complex carbohydrates, sweetened with stevia and xylitol (which are actually good for you), and provide a full spectrum of all-chelated minerals. They also come in a variety of flavors to keep things interesting. They can be purchased at numerous running, cycling, multi-sport, and outdoor outfitter stores. Go online to *hammernutrition.com* to find a dealer near you, or you can order directly from this site.

6. **Build balanced bacterial flora in your intestines for the long term.** It's necessary to nurture and cultivate proper intestinal flora on a daily basis—by eating lactic acid–fermented foods, consuming live culture yogurt, and taking a quality probiotic supplement. Choose the combination that works for you, and stick with it.

7. **Consider using Diamond V XPC.** This fermented yeast culture product has been found to help your body maintain a healthy and balanced immune system, so it can mount an effective defense when necessary but also stop an attack when appropriate. This is critical in autoimmune diseases, where the immune system is "misfiring" by attacking healthy body cells instead of detrimental pathogens. Go to pages 77–79 in the Colorectal Cancer section of this book for full details on this natural, immune-supporting complex.

···············•••••• *Track Your Success!* ··•••••••················

To track your success with this Action Plan, I highly recommend that you record the exact steps you're taking to address your IBD each day, as well as the symptoms you are experiencing at the time, and how you are feeling emotionally.

Putting these details on paper is an excellent way to see what works for you. It's also a great way to document the improvements you're experiencing and just how far you've come using safe, natural solutions to your digestive problem.

Turn to pages 135–136 for sample pages that makes tracking this information simple. Use these pages as your master copy and photocopy more pages to fill in with your details.

Colorectal Cancer

Colorectal cancer—often referred to as colon cancer—occurs when cells in the colon or rectum grow and multiply abnormally, damaging surrounding tissue and interfering with normal colon function.

About 70 percent of colorectal cancers are found in the first six feet of the large intestine, with the balance occurring in the rectum, or last 10 inches of the colon. And it's estimated that 1 in 19 Americans will be diagnosed with this disease at some point in their life.

Risk factors

After age 50, your risk of colorectal cancer increases dramatically—about 90 percent of people with the disease have passed the half-century mark. It affects men, women, and people of all races. And there are often no early signs.

Factors that increase your risk for this cancer are:

- Poor nutrition, especially diets low in pre- and probiotics, vitamin D, selenium, and fiber.

- Diabetes, which increases your risk of colorectal cancer by up to 40 percent.

- Smoking, which may increase your risk of contracting the disease, but most certainly increases your risk of succumbing to it. Research indicates that, once colorectal cancer is diagnosed, smokers face a 30 to 40 percent higher risk of dying from it than non-smokers.

- Alcohol in excess. A glass of wine or beer a day is fine, but anything more than this can increase your risk.

- Inflammatory bowel disease. Ulcerative colitis and Crohn's disease create damage spots in your colon, which makes them vulnerable to DNA mutations and cancer formation.

- Family history. People who have a first-degree family member with colon cancer are more likely to be affected themselves. It's estimated that 20 percent of colon cancers are hereditary.

Symptoms to watch for

Although you can feel perfectly healthy and still have colorectal cancer, there are some common symptoms of the disease. Many, unfortunately, are symptoms shared by many other GI tract conditions, which can delay diagnosis.

However, awareness of symptoms is valuable, if only to encourage you to get regular screenings for colorectal cancer. (More details on this in a minute.)

Symptoms to be aware of are:

- Changes in bowel habits

- Diarrhea

- Bright red or very dark blood in your stool

- Narrow stools

- Gas pains, bloating, feelings of fullness, or cramps

- Vomiting

- Unexplained weight loss

- Chronic fatigue

Rates of colorectal cancer death are falling

The good news about colorectal cancer is that, when detected early, it has a 90 percent cure rate. In the last decade, efforts to promote awareness and prevention techniques have paid off, with colorectal cancer incidence dropping by 22 percent from 1975 to 2000. Similarly colorectal cancer deaths fell by 26 percent during that time period.[29]

Modeling projections made by researchers for the National Cancer Institute found that, if current trends in prevention and detection persist, Americans could see a 36 percent decline in colorectal cancer mortality. And with accelerated cancer control efforts—like trying to get more Americans to adopt favorable health behaviors, such as quitting smoking; a higher use of screening; and enhanced treatment options; there could be a 50 percent reduction in colorectal cancer mortality by the year 2020.[30]

And yet, today, colorectal cancer is still the third leading cause of cancer death for both men and women in America. Clearly, there is more that we can and should do to rein in this lethal disease.

From benign polyp to invasive cancer… the progression of the disease

Colon cancer is largely a reflection of your diet and your lifestyle, which can be protective or damaging to your health. The toxic byproducts of a poor diet, lack of exercise, and unhealthy habits like smoking and excess alcohol, abuse your colon and leave it beleaguered and susceptible to disease.

Our standard American diet, which is woefully low in fiber, antioxidants, and nutrition, while too high in refined flour, sugars, and chemical additives, is a major culprit. Your colon craves fiber, whole foods, and regularity. But when you deliver an unrelenting assault of junk instead, your intestinal cells begin to weaken and change.

It begins with tiny polyps that form in the colon and are almost always benign. But when they are continually exposed to a toxin-laced environment, they can turn cancerous, with corrupted DNA making once-healthy cells grow out of control.

Biotics to the rescue…once again

Not to sound like a broken record, but one of the best ways to preserve and protect colon health is to nurture the colonies of probiotics that reside there. As you now know from my repeated mention of probiotics throughout this book, they take food that we can't digest and feed themselves with it, not only keeping your GI tract running smoothly, but also ensuring that bad bacteria and abnormal growths stay in check.

Prebiotics

Probiotics are powerful intestinal inhabitants, but they can be felled by a diet of junk food or exposure to antibiotics, chronic disease, or stress. Even a hospital stay can wipe them out. This is where prebiotics can help. They'll go a long way to keep your probiotics alive and well. Prebiotics are carbohydrates that your intestinal wall can't absorb, but that your probiotic bacteria thrive on.

Sticking with a diet high in fiber, fruits, and vegetables will give your probiotics the prebiotics they need to stay vital. In addition, the natural sweeteners inulin and oligofructose have turned out to be effective prebiotics. These naturally occurring oligosaccharides, which are chains of non-caloric simple sugar, are produced by plants and are the top food source for specific probiotic strains in your intestines. Natural sources of inulin include artichokes, onions, garlic, agave, and leeks. You can also find inulin and other oligosaccharides in Stonyfield yogurt.

The Humble Food with Superstar Abilities

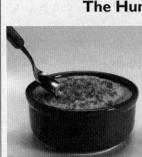

If you're looking for an easy way to help keep your colon healthy and boost your defense against colorectal cancer…look no further than good old fashioned oatmeal for breakfast.

Oats are a humble food, with superstar health-promoting abilities. First of all, they contain both soluble and insoluble fiber—8 grams total in one cup of uncooked oatmeal—which keep your bowels moving and "sweeps them clean" of toxic debris.

But, oats also contain copious amounts of beta-glucan, a fiber-like complex sugar that has been found to be a potent immune system stimulant. Beta-glucan activates the white blood cells known as macrophages and neutrophils. These are the natural killer cells and the "clean-up brigade" that recognize and destroy cancerous tumor cells, accelerate the repair of damaged tissue by removing cellular debris, and trigger additional components of the immune system.[31]

So eat more oats. They're one of the few nutrient-rich foods that you can still easily find that haven't been contaminated, overly processed, or denatured.

When you buy oats, don't get instant oatmeal, which has already been partially cooked and often contains sugar, salt, or other ingredients. "Old-fashioned oats" take a little longer to cook, but the 15 minutes will be well worth the wait. Also, I wouldn't buy oats in large quantities. The beneficial fats in oats can go rancid with time. Fresh oats should smell fresh. Generally, if they are in an airtight container in a cool, dry, dark area, you can expect them to last about two months.

Synbiotics

Pro- and prebiotics together are called synbiotics, a term coined to describe the synergistic effects of taking them together. The first human study of synbiotics confirmed that they exhibit anticancer effects. They make the cells in your colon healthier and more stable, with better immunity and fewer cancerous DNA mutations.

The European SynCan (short for Synbiotics and Cancer Prevention) project uses research to determine whether prebiotics, probiotics, and synbiotics can reduce the risk of colorectal cancer, which is now the most common form of cancer in the European Union.

Researchers found that synbiotics improved intestinal flora, reduced toxin damage, and changed gene expression in both the polyp and cancer groups. This indicates the critical importance of using pre- and probiotics together for their overall GI health benefits as well as their colorectal cancer prevention benefits.

Preventative health from an unlikely source

Another preventative health tool for those at risk for colorectal cancer comes from an unlikely source—an animal feed supplement manufacturer.

A few years ago I got a very interesting call about a company called Diamond V Mills located in Cedar Rapids, Iowa, which makes an animal feed supplement from a fermented yeast culture. Supplements like this aren't unusual. Numerous companies manufacture and sell either baker's yeast or yeast cultures to add to animal feeds. Diamond V has been doing so for over 60 years. This call, though, had to do with the health of the employees at Diamond V, not the animals feeding on their products.

When checking through health claim records, Diamond V found that their plant workers, who came into contact with the yeast products, weren't getting sick. Their support staff, however, took sick leave at rates that were comparable to most companies across the country. After accounting for all the other possible factors, it appeared the improved health of those in the production plant could be traced to their repeated exposure to the fermented yeast culture dust in the production plant.

Subsequent interviews revealed, time and time again, that an employee's health picture often changed dramatically after coming to work at Diamond V Mills. Some, despite experiencing yearly flu and colds in the past, reported they had not had either in the years since they started work at the plant. Some hadn't experienced a cold, flu, or other infection in 25 years. Others reported improvement in gastrointestinal health, chronic allergy conditions, autoimmune problems, and numerous other conditions after starting work at the plant.

Researchers then began to take a closer look at the effects yeast cultures might have on humans. Their findings were amazing, to say the least. After more research and product development, the company came up with a more concentrated product for humans and it has now been associated with a wide variety of very significant health benefits.[32]

Immune function on the rise

One important research finding was that, with continued use of concentrated yeast culture, natural killer (NK) cell activity increased fourfold. These cells are your immune system's first line of defense against invading pathogens or cancer cells. This increased efficiency allowed the immune system to perform at superior levels with fewer NK cells—sparing the body the stress and expenditure of having to produce more NK cells.

It also improved the ratio of immune helper cells to suppressor cells. In the simplest terms, helper cells are crucial in coordinating the response of the immune system to pathogens. They activate other immune cells and stimulate the production of antibodies. Suppressor cells, on the other hand, stop an attack and help maintain a balance so your immune system doesn't "over-react." Individuals taking the yeast culture also exhibited higher levels of antibodies, indicating their immune systems were more effective.

And what I believe to be one of the most important findings of all has to do with levels of what's called immunoglobulin A (IgA). Our first line of defense against ingested pathogens is a protective mucus layer. IgA is an antibody found in the mucosal lining of the respiratory and digestive tracts and is an indicator of mucosal barrier strength. The research showed that ingesting (even if through inhalation) this fermented yeast culture resulted in astoundingly higher levels of IgA, indicating a much stronger mucus layer to protect the body against pathogens.

Simple health from a complex compound

Like many other natural products, yeast cultures are very complex—and there are unquestionably dozens of components that contribute to its efficacy. The compounds in the human product developed by Diamond V included some surprises:

- **Selenium**, a powerful antioxidant. Insufficient selenium in the diet allows viruses to mutate, which helps explain why we see most of the flu viruses arising from parts of the world with selenium-deficient soils.

- **Squalene**, a steroid precursor and powerful immune-boosting component normally found in only a few species of sharks and a few plants.

- **Resveratrol**, one of the true "anti-aging" compounds, which is normally found in grape skins and red wine.

- **All the primary minerals, trace minerals, amino acids, and several B vitamins**, as well as other beneficial compounds normally found only in foods like blueberries and green tea.

In addition, the lab tests revealed that the yeast culture has over three times the antioxidant capacity of any known food. The oxygen radical absorbance capacity (ORAC) of the product was shown to be 614—almost four times the highest ORAC-value food, black raspberries, which have a value of 164. ORAC is an important measure of antioxidant levels in foods and other substances. It reflects the ability of a substance to eliminate oxygen free radicals.

Proven safety

Extensive toxicology studies conducted on this cultured yeast product show it to be nontoxic and safe. Even at extremely high dosages, there has never been any indication of side effects. It has also been tested for over 139 of the most common pesticides and toxic residues, and it contains none of them. Additional tests have been performed to determine if it interferes with over-the-counter or prescription medications, and it doesn't.

I'm sure one concern for many people has to be the fact that the product is a yeast culture. Individuals bothered with systemic infections from the yeast *Candida albicans* are hesitant about including any yeast products in their diet. Yeast infections have been linked to numerous chronic health problems.

It's important to remember, however, that this product is a dried, fermented yeast culture. As opposed to live yeast, this culture contains the fermented metabolites of a once-live colony of yeast, as well as the dead yeast itself and the residue of the medium it was grown on. It doesn't transfer live yeast organisms to your GI tract, but instead facilitates and increases the growth of the existing beneficial bacterial flora.

Most everyone has *Candida albicans* and dozens of other potential pathogens living in their lower GI tract, but few of those people go on to experience any problems because their level of beneficial bacteria is sufficient to keep the pathogens in check.

Gut-level benefits

Components of this product work as a prebiotic to feed the beneficial bacteria in your gut. The yeast culture also provides its own, very potent metabolites that inhibit the growth of harmful viruses, bacteria, fungi, and other pathogens.

Very minute levels—as small as one part per billion—of this product have been shown to totally inhibit the growth of *E. coli*, the bacteria most commonly associated with food poisoning. It also completely stopped the growth of *Candida tropicalis*, which is the second most commonly encountered pathogen and a major cause of blood poisoning (septicemia)—particularly among individuals with diabetes, leukemia, or lymphoma.

The combination of dead yeast and metabolites in this yeast culture also increases mass in the gastrointestinal tract, and improves fiber and protein digestion by supplying a long list of various nutrients and enzymes.

Prevention rather than a cure

One of the strongest attributes of this product is the fact that it balances the immune system rather than acting as an immune stimulant. (This is why I recommend it for those suffering with IBD autoimmune disorders as well as those concerned with colorectal cancer.)

Since it's not a stimulant, it wouldn't be used as a "treatment" for some acute problem like a cold or flu. Instead, it's something that can be taken continuously to prevent a cold, flu, or other infection from happening in the first place. It's a maintenance-type product that has a history of being safe and effective for long-term use.

Getting the yeast

Diamond V Mills has a few different cultured yeast products for animals; the formulations are essentially the same except for their concentration. The most concentrated, and the one I use and recommend, is called Diamond V XPC. It's based on the yeast *Saccharomyces cerevisiae*. The medium on which the yeast is grown consists of processed grain byproducts, roughage products, cane molasses, malt, and corn syrup. These natural sugars are necessary to feed the yeast.

The yeast they use is also commonly referred to as baker's yeast or brewer's yeast. It is one of the most researched yeasts and has been used for centuries for making bread, beer (particularly ales...my favorite), and wine. Diamond V reportedly utilizes a proprietary technique to both grow and dry the yeast, which helps maintain its health-promoting benefits.

When the company discovered that cultured yeast could benefit humans as well as animals, it formed a subsidiary called Embria Health Sciences to sell the newly developed product under the name EpiCor. Although the improved immune health I've discussed is a direct result of ingesting the products created for animals, the company literature says that EpiCor and Diamond V XPC are somewhat different.

For one, the company says the drying process is different so the product retains more of its antioxidant capability. From the company's product specification sheets I've obtained, it appears that EpiCor may also have a higher protein level.

A significant difference from the company's point of view is that EpiCor is made in a food-grade facility, while the Diamond V XPC products are made in a feed-grade plant. I'm sure that matters to the FDA, but it doesn't matter to me.

EpiCor has the FDA safety status of Generally Recognized As Safe (GRAS). Diamond V doesn't, but then products for animals generally don't. The approval process is lengthy and expensive, and not necessary for animal feed. Nevertheless, both are obviously safe, nontoxic, pesticide free, and non-mutagenic. They both have the same reported shelf life: a minimum of 24 months from the date of manufacture.

The biggest difference I see between the two products, however, is the price. A 30-day supply of EpiCor (consisting of thirty 500 mg capsules) sells for anywhere from about $20 to $50. A 50-pound bag of Diamond V XPC sells at feed stores for anywhere from $1.50 to $1.75 a pound.

Getting the right amount

Recommended dosages for Diamond V XPC vary significantly depending on the size of the animal. The company's literature obviously doesn't provide dosages for human use, but, if you use body weight as the determining factor, the dosage for an adult human would be in the ballpark of 2 to 3 grams, which translates to about ¾ to 1 teaspoon a day.

At the time the company first noticed the effect the product had on humans, they carried out tests to see approximately how much was being taken in daily by the workers. Diamond V used the results of these tests to determine the dosage of EpiCor to be a half gram per day. Based on this dosage figure, a daily dose of EpiCor, from the least expensive supplier I could find, would run about 66 cents.

The dosage of XPC that's equivalent to half a gram of EpiCor is about 3 grams. This daily dosage, at the highest price I could find for XPC, would cost only 2 cents a day.

I'm going into such detail because I don't see how anyone can pass on this deal. I've personally never seen a better bargain when it comes to balancing your immune system. If you utilize the XPC product, you can help give your body some of the best protection ever documented for 2 cents a day. This is a product my dad would certainly call "cheap insurance."

I'm sure the company won't like the comparisons I'm making, but the facts are there. And for several reasons they can't recommend that humans use XPC. But it wasn't EpiCor that bestowed all the end benefits on the employees at Diamond V Mills; it was the lesser-concentrated animal products. And those products have been used successfully on all types of animals for over 63 years without incident. Like it or not, we too are animals.

Where to get your supply

If you'd rather not mess with getting a 50-pound bag of XPC or prefer the convenience of taking a premade capsule, you can get EpiCor from quite a few suppliers, including Vitamin Research Products at *vrp.com* or 1-800-877-2447; and Healthy Origins, at *healthyorigins.com* or 1-888-228-6650.

If you're like me, however, and just can't pass up the deal of spending just 2 cents per day for this amazing immune health protector, then you can get XPC from Wholesale Feeds in Marion, Iowa. They can't take Internet orders yet, but you can call them at 1-319-377-5528. (Remember that the product is sold for animal use, so don't ask them questions about use for humans.) You can also try your local feed store. If they don't have the product, ask if they can order it for you.

Some people may not think XPC tastes that good. If you are one and have the time and inclination, you can make your own capsules. Empty capsules and capsule-filling machines are available at many local health food stores or from Penn Herb Company at *pennherb.com* or 1-800-523-9971.

Personally, I find it much easier to simply put the powder in my protein shake each morning, or just take the ¾ to 1 teaspoon of the powder and put it directly in my mouth. The grainy, yeast flavor reminds me of my days as a child growing up on a farm and, frankly, I like it.

More solutions for a healthy colon

While pre- and probiotics, as well as Diamond V XPC, can help set the stage for colon health, there are other nutrients that can help protect your colon health and play an important role in the treatment protocol for colorectal cancer. These are:

- **B vitamins.** Scientists have found a compelling connection between reduced folate levels in the blood and an increased risk of colorectal cancer. A good B-complex or a high-quality multi-nutrient will give you the necessary levels. **Note:** If you are taking Diamond V XPC, you are already getting small amounts of some B vitamins.

- **Vitamin E.** A 10-year study has shown a 50 percent reduction in colorectal cancer in individuals who take 200 IU of vitamin E daily. Make sure to take a source of E that includes mixed tocopherols, both gamma and d-alpha, and, ideally, tocotrienols.

- **Vitamin D.** Your body manufactures this essential vitamin from direct exposure to sunlight or you can get vitamin D from your diet. Be sure to spend at least

15–20 minutes outdoors every day in the sunshine and, for insurance, take from 1,000 to 3,000 mg vitamin D daily.

- **Calcium.** This mineral is well known for its bone health benefits, but several preliminary studies have shown that calcium supplementation also helps reduce the risk of colorectal cancer and precancerous polyps. In addition, calcium may bind to bile acid, reducing the harm it causes your colon. Take at least 700 mg a day.

- **Bromelain.** This plant-derived enzyme aids in protein digestion and reduces the pain, gas, and bowel frequency associated with poor digestion. The healthier your digestion, the more efficiently your colon works. Take 500–1,000 mg a day, with meals.

- **Resveratrol**, a naturally occurring compound found in grapes, may help protect against the growth and proliferation of colon cancer cells. In fact, a study published in *Cancer Letters* found that resveratrol reduced the growth rate of colon cancer cells by an amazing 70 percent. I recommend 200 mg, standardized to at least 8 percent total resveratrol, mixed with flavonoids for better bioavailability. **Note:** Because resveratrol has anticoagulation effects, consult your doctor before using it if you have a blood-clotting condition.

- **Selenium.** This powerful antioxidant has been found to inhibit cancer in animal studies. Additional research indicates that selenium shows promise in colorectal cancer prevention in humans. If you are at risk for colon cancer, start with a dosage of 600 mcg per day for 6 to 9 months, and then continue at 200 to 300 mcg per day.

- **Garlic.** Research has shown that eating 1–2 cloves daily of raw or cooked garlic decreases the chance of colon cancer by 30 percent, and stomach cancer by 50 percent.

- **Ground flaxseed.** This is a great source of soluble fiber, as well as mucilage and lubricants, which both bulks up and softens your stool, making it easier to move through your intestines. And its lignans give you the added bonus of enhanced immune response. Just blend 4–6 tablespoons per day into shakes or cereal.

Get screened!

Early detection of colon polyps is essential for preventing colorectal cancer. And early detection of cancerous tumors before they can spread to your body's lymph nodes or other organs is absolutely critical for survival. Yet, half of the 80 million people over the age of 50 have never been screened for colon cancer.

This is definitely one case where ignorance is NOT bliss. It can literally be the difference between life and death. In 37 percent of people diagnosed with colorectal cancer, the cancer is confined to superficial cell layers of the colon, which is a "best-case scenario," or extends through the intestinal wall but hasn't reached the lymph nodes. The survival rate in these cases of early detection is 90 percent.

But nearly two-thirds of people diagnosed with this form of cancer find that it has already progressed through the wall of the colon or rectum into the lymph nodes, or has already spread to other organs, such as the liver or lungs. In these cases, the survival rate is just 5 percent.

It's a startling difference with a message that's crystal clear: Preventive screening pays. So, here are some details to help you get the best screening, with as little worry, discomfort, and expense as possible.

Smear test

There are a variety of screening tests for colorectal cancer and the simplest one is a smear test or fecal occult blood test. This is when your doctor takes a small amount of stool gathered during a digital rectal exam and smears it on a card with a reagent on it. The reagent will turn color if there's any blood in the stool, which is one of the classic signs of colorectal cancer. This test is something your doctor can perform at your annual physical exam, with little additional time, cost, or discomfort.

Unfortunately, just-released research from the U.S. Centers for Disease Control and Prevention indicate that the single sample fecal occult blood test missed detecting cancers and precancerous polyps 95 percent of the time. For this reason, the more accurate home-based fecal occult blood test (see below) is the one recommended in national testing guidelines.[33]

Home use kit

Another way to test for hidden blood in the stool is with a home-use kit. There is one I recommend that makes the process simple, reliable, and virtually hassle free. It's called the EZ Detect test and it's clinically proven and FDA approved.

You don't have to handle any stool with this kit, which makes the process a lot more agreeable. Instead, you simply drop a biodegradable test paper into the toilet bowl after a bowel movement, and wait for two minutes. That's it. If there's blood in the stool, a cross on the test tissue will turn blue-green to let you know.

One test kit contains five test tissues, one to test your clean toilet water, to make sure nothing in it turns the test falsely positive. It should not turn color. The next three you use for your next three bowel movements. Testing three times gives you highly accurate results. The fifth and final tissue is a positive control, where you drop in the tissue in clean water, add the positive control chemical to the water, and watch the cross turn color. This helps you understand and validate that the test is working and that you got dependable results. **Note:** Do not take this test if you are suffering from constipation and can't produce a fecal sample or if you're experiencing menstrual or hemorrhoidal bleeding, because of the possibility of a false reading. Wait for a better time.

A major advantage with this testing method is that you don't have to change your diet or stop your supplements. All other testing methods advise some form of dietary restriction, such as to temporarily stop eating red meat, broccoli, vitamin C, and others.

Amazingly enough, EZ Detect is affordable, and most insurance programs, including Medicare, pay for some colorectal screening. You don't need a prescription for it. You can order directly from *ezdetect.com* or by calling 1-800-854-3002. It costs just $7.99 per test kit, plus $3.65 shipping in the U.S.

Colorectal screening guidelines established in 1997 in the U.S. say that simply performing a yearly fecal blood test could cut colorectal cancer deaths by one-third. And now that the EZ Detect kit makes it so simple, there's really no excuse not to get this screening each and every year.

Colonoscopy

The gold standard of colon cancer screening is still the colonoscopy. It's a visual exam of the entire colon and allows for the removal of accessible polyps. It's a procedure that I have discussed briefly earlier in this book, and it's a must for everyone over the age of 50. If you have any risk factor for colorectal cancer, you should start this screening earlier. Consult your doctor to determine the best time.

If you get a "clean bill of health" after your colonoscopy (and aren't in any high risk categories for colon cancer), then you should get repeat colonoscopies every 7–10 years. If your colonoscopy reveals polyps or other precancerous cells, or if you are in a high risk category, your doctor will likely recommend a shorter time between colonoscopies—probably every 2–5 years.

Ease your worries

The thought of undergoing a colonoscopy is no doubt worrisome. I believe this is one of the biggest reasons that so few people get this screening as advised. But, knowing what to expect is a great way to allay those fears. Once you have details in hand, I'm sure you'll agree that colonoscopies are nothing to fear and certainly nothing to avoid—especially given their huge health payoff.

First of all, colonoscopies have come a long way in the last decade. Better, smaller, more flexible instruments with minute camera optics make the process much less invasive and much more comfortable. And most of the time, colonoscopies are performed with the patient under sedative medication, which means you will be feeling calm, serene, and just vaguely aware of the procedure as it happens. Most people don't feel any pain or even remember the test, and can go home a little while after the procedure is complete. On average, the total time you'll spend at the medical facility for your colonoscopy is about three hours.

Preparation is the key to success

One of the most important factors leading to a successful colonoscopy is how well you do your part to prepare your colon for the procedure. This is because the better your colon is cleared of all fecal matter, the better view your doctor will have of your entire colon.

By all accounts, the preparation phase is the most unpleasant part of the colonos-copy process. It takes much longer than the colonoscopy itself, and involves purging your bowels, which isn't fun by any measure.

But, you can work with your doctor to select the best preparation method for you and you can take steps on your own to minimize the unpleasantries.

Diet leading up to bowel prep day

Your doctor will give you specific directions, but generally, during the 24 hours before your bowel-cleansing day and up to a few hours before the colonoscopy itself, you won't eat solids and will drink only clear liquids, like water, broths, lemon-lime soda or seltzer, and ginger ale. You can have Jell-O and suck on hard candy, but make sure they don't contain any red, blue, or purple coloring. Your doctor may also advise you to avoid insoluble fiber in the form of nuts and seeds for a day or so prior to your clear liquid regimen.

Four common options for bowel cleansing

In order to clear your bowels as completely as possible to give your doctor the very best view during your colonoscopy, you'll need to have some purgative help. This usually comes in one of four forms. Work with your doctor to choose the method that will do the most thorough job with the least amount of stress.

Bowel Prep Type	Process	Good-to-Know Details
Polyethylene glycol (PEG) Sold under the names: CoLyte, GoLytely, NuLytely, TriLyte	This preparation consists of a gallon jug with a powder mix inside. You fill the jug with water to make a drink out of the powder and then drink one 8-ounce glass of the mixture every 10 minutes until you've finished the entire gallon or your eliminations are clear. After the first few glasses, bowel evacuations will begin. Many people find that their evacuations are totally clear before the gallon of PEG is gone. An alternate approach is to divide the jug into quarters and drink ¾ the night before the colonoscopy and ¼ the morning of.	PEG solutions are electrolyte balanced and work by introducing a large amount of fluid to force out waste from your bowel. They taste salty and the large fluid volume can cause nausea and bloating, and sometimes vomiting and cramping. You may want to have some anti-nausea measures at the ready, like ginger root capsules. Take one to two 650 mg capsules every eight hours as needed. Available from Penn Herb Co. (1-800-523-9971).
Oral sodium phosphate (OSP) solution Sold under the names: Fleet Accu-Prep, Fleet Phospho-soda, EZ-Prep	Take 2 doses of the OSP solution with at least 8 ounces of clear fluids, about 10 to 12 hours apart. Follow your dose with 16 more ounces of clear fluids.	OSP solutions work by pulling water into your bowels to cleanse them. Doesn't require the liquid volume needed with PEG solutions, but can lead to dehydration or electrolyte imbalances if you don't get sufficient fluids during the process. May cause kidney injury.
Oral sodium phosphate (OSP) tablets Sold under the names: OsmoPrep, Visicol	With OsmoPrep (a newer formulation), on the evening before your colonoscopy, you take 4 tablets with 8 ounces of clear fluids every 15 minutes for an hour and a quarter (20 tablets total). Then take 12 more tablets in the same way 3–5 hours before your colonoscopy. With Visicol, on the evening before your colonoscopy, you take 7 doses in 15-minute intervals. For the first 6 doses, you take 3 tablets together, and for the last dose you take 2 tablets (20 tablets total). The next morning, 3–5 hours before your colonoscopy, repeat the dosing (3 tablets for 6 doses, and then 2 tablets for 1 dose in 15-minute intervals for a total of 20 tablets).	OSP tablets work in the same way as OSP solution, and have the same pros and cons. May cause kidney injury.
Laxatives Sold as magnesium citrate, bisacodyl	Laxatives are usually used in conjunction with a lower-volume PEG solution, like HalfLytely, which requires you to drink about half the liquid of other PEG solutions. They are also used along with OSP tablets.	Although usually used in conjunction with another bowel preparation, magnesium citrate can be used alone.

Source: The Harvard Medical School Family Health Guide [34]

Six Tried-and-True Tips for Worry-Free Colonoscopy Prep

Here are some tips to help ensure your bowel prep is a success with minimum stress.

1. **Get your colonoscopy preparation instructions from your doctor well in advance of the procedure date.** Read them over and call your doctor with any questions.

2. **Pick up the preparations prescribed by your doctor and make sure you have all the things required for mixing and drinking on hand.** And get a box of medicated wet wipes with aloe and vitamin E to keep cleanup soothing, not irritating.

3. **Make arrangements so you can have the privacy you want.** Clear your schedule and get coverage for the kids or relatives under your care.

4. **Add variety to your clear liquids.** Staying adequately hydrated is essential during your bowel prep, but sticking with plain water can get boring. So keep other clear liquids on hand, like ginger ale, broths, or lemon-lime soda or seltzer. Popsicles, Jell-O and even Italian ice (if not colored with red, blue, or purple dye) will help at taste and a little texture, too.

5. **Wear loose, easy-on easy-off clothing.** Sometimes the urge to purge comes quickly, and you won't want to be bothered with difficult buttons or zippers. Keep it simple with sweat pants, elastic waist shorts, or something similar.

6. **Keep things interesting.** You'll need to stay near...or perhaps in...your bathroom for most of the day, so make it as comfortable and interesting as possible. Bring a book and some fun magazines to read. Laptop? Set it up nearby so you can stay connected during your clear-out. Cell phone? Have it handy. And soothing music or aromatherapy oils can help you stay calm, cool, and collected.

PART II

The actual process

During a colonoscopy, the doctor guides a thin, flexible tube with a tiny camera through the colon to check for, and when necessary, remove abnormalities, including cancerous and precancerous growths.

On average, it takes seven minutes for a doctor to guide the colonoscopy device to the top of the colon and another six minutes to withdraw it as he or she evaluates the inside of the colon. Pausing to remove an abnormal growth takes about four extra minutes, on average.

When you're looking for a doctor to perform your exam, ask candidates how long they take to withdraw the scope and evaluate the colon. A new study conducted at the University of Illinois College of Medicine and published in the *New England Journal of Medicine* found that physicians who normally took more than the six-minute average to complete the examination identified up to four times as many abnormal growths compared to those who rushed through the procedure.

CT colonography

Computerized tomography (CT) scanning is a newer technology used to screen for colon polyps and cancer. It's also used in cases of ulcerative colitis or Crohn's disease to evaluate colon health, and I mentioned it in the IBD section of this book. But here are a few more details.

CT scanning combines highly sensitive X-ray equipment with sophisticated computers to produce cross-sectional pictures of the inside of the body. In the case of a CT colonography, it's the colon that's being pictured.

Just as you do for a traditional colonoscopy, you need to clean out your colon prior to a CT colonography. You also need to take small amounts of barium and iodinated liquids just prior to the procedure to help the radiologist get better pictures so your doctor can more accurately analyze them.

How the CT scan works

The CT scanner looks like a large box-shaped machine with a hole in the center, where the examination bed that you lie on can slide into. During the scan, you will be asked to lie on your back, stomach, and side.

As the CT scans, multiple X-ray beams and a set of X-ray detectors rotate around you as your examination bed moves through the scanner. This technique is called helical or spiral CT. The cross-sectional pictures of your colon are then fed into a computer that produces detailed, three-dimensional models of your abdominal area. It gives your doctor views of your colon as if he were looking at it with a traditional scope…yet it's a simulation. For this reason, a CT colonography is often referred to as a "virtual" colonoscopy.

Advantages of the CT colonography

One advantage of this technology is that it's less invasive than a traditional colonoscopy, which uses a scope inserted in your rectum and guided through your entire colon. As such, it has a lower risk of colon perforation than conventional colonoscopy does (although this procedural risk is rare even in conventional colonoscopies).

Be aware, though, that doctors conducting a CT colonography will place a small tube several inches into your rectum, which pumps carbon dioxide gas into the colon to distend it and eliminate any folds or wrinkles in the surface that could obscure polyps from the doctor's view. The carbon dioxide can create uncomfortable passing of gas for up to a few days after the procedure.

Another advantage of the CT colonography is that it's faster than a traditional colonoscopy. In fact, CT scanners can process large parts of the body in just seconds and the entire examination usually only takes 15 minutes.

This minimally invasive screening alternative is an excellent choice for people who have risk of complications during a traditional colonoscopy—such as those on blood thinners or who have severe breathing issues. It's also helpful for ill or elderly patients who may not tolerate the sedation required for a traditional colonoscopy. Finally, it's a good choice for people who have a narrowed or obstructed colon that would make using a colonoscopy scope difficult.

A DNA test alternative

If you're unable to undergo a colonoscopy, there is an alternative for you to consider. It's called ColoSure, and it's a new DNA home test. It actually analyzes the DNA in your stool to determine whether there's evidence of genetic mutations that occur in all cancer cells. When a cancer grows in the colon, it sheds cells into the stool.

ColoSure tests your stool sample for 23 DNA markers associated with colorectal cancer and pre-cancerous polyps. Although it's safe and simple, it's somewhat expensive at $399 per kit. For more information, go to *dnadirect.com*.

⫸ Your Action Plan for Preventing Colorectal Cancer ⫸

As I've emphasized many times, prevention is the key when it comes to colorectal cancer. And I've outlined numerous tools and techniques to consider for keeping your bowels healthy and functioning optimally, and for keeping colorectal cancer at bay. I'll recap them here, as well as add a few more tips to follow in your Action Plan.

1. **Eat a healthy, balanced diet high in fiber and low in sugar and saturated fat.** Emphasize raw, organic fruits and vegetables, especially cruciferous vegetables, like broccoli, bok choy, Brussels sprouts, cress, kale, radish, turnip, kohlrabi, cabbage, and cauliflower. These antioxidant-rich vegetables have been found to decrease the effects of cancer-causing chemicals. Also, drink pure, clean water to help prevent GI enzyme depletion and to support healthy GI structure and function.

2. **Avoid chemicals, toxins, and known carcinogens** as much as possible, including alcohol and red meat. Research indicates that just one serving of red meat per day is associated with a 50 percent increase in colorectal cancer risk. And, of course, don't smoke.

3. **Take a digestive enzyme supplement** to restore enzymes depleted by processed foods, caffeine, alcohol, and stress. These are available in most health food stores or you can contact Progressive Laboratories for their product, Digestin #987 (*progressivelabs.com* or 1-800-527-9512).

4. **Start on Diamond V XPC or EpiCor to boost your immune system** and fortify your overall good health. At less than 2 cents a day, Diamond V XPC is probably the best value in anticancer protection ever. You can get XPC from Wholesale Feeds in Marion, Iowa (1-319-377-5528) and you can order

EpiCor from Vitamin Research Products (*vrp.com* or 1-800-877-2447) and Healthy Origins (*healthyorigins.com* or 1-888-228-6650).

5. **Consider the colon health-supporting supplements and dietary nutrients** outlined for you on pages 73–76.

6. **Fortify your gut with prebiotics and probiotics**. Prebiotics are plentiful in artichokes, onions, garlic, agave, and leeks. Eat more lactic acid–fermented foods and live culture yogurt for your probiotics. Prebiotics and probiotics can be found together in supplement form in a product called a symbiotic. While these products are usually not labeled as symbiotics, there are plenty that function as symbiotics. I recommend Inu-Max (*www.inumax.com* or 1-877-812-5716) and Now Foods Gr8-Dophilus (widely available).

7. **Engage in regular exercise.** It improves your digestive health, cardiovascular health, and mental health. It will also help you maintain a healthy weight— another important means of keeping health issues, including cancer, at bay. Research shows that exercise is directly connected with prevention of breast, prostate, and colon cancers. Start off your exercise routine slowly—about 10–15 minutes a day. As you become more fit, increase the time and intensity of your workout, so that eventually, you are exercising 30–60 minutes at least five days a week.

8. **De-stress.** Consistently high stress levels make you more susceptible to cancer and other chronic diseases. Plus, unresolved stress has been linked to certain bowel conditions that can be precursors to colorectal cancer. Try relaxation techniques mentioned in Part I of this book, such as yoga or meditation. And don't be afraid to seek the advice of a counselor, if necessary.

9. **Get regular screening.** This is of utmost importance. Work with your doctor to select the most appropriate screening option for you, and then DO IT! Remember, the best screening is the one that gets done.

• • • • • • • • • • • • • • • • • • • • *Track Your Success!* **• • • • • • • • • • • • • • • • • • • •**

To track your success with this Action Plan, I suggest that you record the exact steps you're taking to address your colon health.

Putting these details on paper is an excellent way to see what works for you. It's also a great way to document the improvements you're experiencing and to let you know when you need to schedule your regular colon cancer screening.

The tracking sheet I've recommended for other digestive health concerns may not work in this case. Here, you're taking preventative health steps rather than addressing a particular condition with troubling symptoms. A simple spiral notebook where you can jot down your "to do's" for keeping your colon healthy and checking each one off as you do it will probably do the trick.

When colorectal cancer is your reality

There is probably no other word in the English language that strikes as much fear into the heart of so many as the word "cancer." Despite decades of research and scientific advancement, conventional cancer treatments—surgery, chemotherapy, and radiation—can hardly be called successful.

This is especially true of chemotherapy, which tries to target fast reproducing cancer cells, yet causes a tremendous amount of collateral damage in the process. It leaves your body weakened and vulnerable, and far less able to effectively mount its own natural defense against the attack of cancer.

Yet, as is the case with most any cancer, if you're diagnosed with colorectal cancer, your doctor will likely recommend one of the three standard treatment options, or perhaps a combination of the three.

One bright point related to colorectal cancer is that, if your cancer is diagnosed before any tumor has penetrated your bowel wall, then surgery to remove the tumor often results in a cure.

However, if your tumor has spread through the bowel wall, then a more aggressive approach with radiation, a chemotherapeutic agent, or both will likely be considered. Work closely with your doctor to find the combination that provides the best possible outcome for your particular situation.

But don't let your body take the abuse of both cancer cells and conventional treatments without giving it the extra support it needs to fight back to good health. The building blocks for creating a healthy digestive system foundation that I outlined for you in Part I of this book and the recommendations I made for preventing colorectal cancer will all help.

But there are other profoundly effective solutions direct from Mother Nature that can help you support your immune system in this battle for your life and nourish your entire body so it can not only withstand the negative effects of cancer treatment, but also move forward in the journey to regain long-term good health.

Following are three of the best that you should know about.

Avemar

One exciting natural cancer therapy that I want to bring to your attention is a fermented wheat germ extract from Hungary known as Avemar. Since its development in the mid-90s, there have been over 100 studies on Avemar demonstrating its effectiveness in the treatment of cancer.

A myriad of possibilities

A discovery like Avemar would be considered promising if it were effective in the treatment of just one or two forms of cancer, but it goes far beyond that. What's so amazing about Avemar is that it doesn't appear to be specific to any one particular type of cancer. Instead, both in the laboratory and in all follow-up animal and human studies, Avemar has been effective against all cancer cell lines tested, including colorectal cancer.

One controlled study involved 170 people with colorectal cancer. Researchers contrasted the effects of using Avemar plus conventional "standard of care" treatments—surgery, radiation, and chemotherapy—with the results of conventional treatments alone. The benefits of adding Avemar were remarkable. The addition of Avemar resulted in an 82 percent reduction in new tumor recurrences, a 67 percent reduction in metastases, and a 62 percent reduction in deaths.[35]

Another study involved 30 patients with advanced colorectal cancer. All the patients underwent surgery, and 12 of them began taking Avemar. At the end of the nine-month observation period, there was no disease progression in any of the patients on Avemar. However, in the control group, three patients had died from the disease and another had developed metastatic tumors.[36]

A third study involved 34 patients suffering from advanced adenocarcinoma of the rectum or lower colon. After corrective surgery, 17 received the conventional treatment and the other 17 received conventional treatment plus Avemar. Forty-six months later, those on the Avemar had significantly longer survival rates.[37]

And much, much more

In addition to studies on Avemar's effects on the course of colorectal cancer, there have been similar studies related to melanoma and breast cancer, also with positive results. And there have been in vitro studies of cell cultures as well as animal studies involving implanted tumors that have shown Avemar can be effective against cell lines from lymphoma, leukemia, lung cancer, oral cavity cancer, and pancreatic cancer.

Perhaps the most research activity is in Hungary where Avemar was developed. With the full support of the Hungarian government and the medical community, Avemar has been used in Hungary for over a decade to help successfully treat cancer patients. In fact, it's officially classified there as "a medical nutrient for cancer patients."

How does Avemar work?

Avemar works through several different mechanisms. One of its most unique benefits, however, is its ability to inhibit glucose metabolism in cancer cells.

Every form of cancer cell requires large amounts of glucose—10 to 50 times more than normal healthy cells. Glucose conversion produces nucleic acids and proteins, the building materials that a cancer requires to continue growing. This process is referred to as the "Warburg effect."

Research at UCLA has demonstrated that Avemar reduces glucose flow into cancer cells, which inhibits their ability to produce additional nucleic acids and to proliferate. In fact, in the presence of Avemar compounds, cancer cells actually begin to produce substances that inhibit cell division and stimulate programmed cell death within the tumor. In other words, Avemar triggers cancer cell "suicide." And it does so without any toxic side effects or damage to normal, healthy cells.

Safe and effective

Avemar's safety has been studied extensively in cell lines, animals, and humans and no adverse effects have been identified. Researchers actually compared Avemar's toxicological profile to that of bread. (Though the product is made from only the germ part of wheat, the manufacturer has included a caution for people who are sensitive to gluten.)

But Avemar isn't just free from adverse effects. It also has the added benefit of being able to protect your body's cells against the toxic effects of conventional cancer therapies. In all of the studies where Avemar was used in conjunction with conventional therapies, not only were those therapies significantly more effective, but the patients experienced considerably less frequent and severe nausea, fatigue, weight loss, and depression. Additionally, the patients' immune systems recovered more rapidly.[38]

Works against cancer metastasis, too

Another very significant finding, consistent in practically all of the Avemar studies, is that Avemar is particularly effective at reducing metastasis, or the spreading of the cancer to other sites throughout the body.

The capability of your immune system has a big influence on whether your cancer will spread. And research has shown that Avemar can dramatically boost the response and effectiveness of the immune system—even when it's been compromised by cancer and cancer therapy.[39] That's why I believe that Avemar is useful at any stage of the cancer process—even in the more advanced stages, when the body's immune system is severely impaired.

Getting and taking Avemar

Avemar is produced in Budapest, Hungary, by Biromedicina. In the United States, the product is being sold under the name AvéUltra instead of Avemar, but otherwise it's exactly the same. It's available through The Harmony Company (*theharmonyco.com* or 1-888-809-1241).

AvéUltra comes in convenient individual packets, each containing 5.5 grams of Avemar—the recommended single daily dose for a 70 kilogram (154 pound) adult, and the amount given in the clinical studies.

You should mix each packet with 4 ounces of cold water and then drink it either an hour before or an hour after a meal. Additionally, you should drink your AvéUltra and water mix either two hours before or two hours after taking any other drugs or dietary supplements—particularly vitamin C, which some studies indicate may dampen the effectiveness of Avemar.

Modified citrus pectin

Another natural product has repeatedly shown promise in preventing cancer metastases. It's a form of pectin—a complex carbohydrate that's commonly used for gelling jams, jellies, and yogurt. Pectin is found in practically all plants. It's the structural fiber that helps give the cell walls of the plant their shape and strength. Years ago, when fiber was a leading health topic and hot-selling supplement, there was considerable interest in pectin, particularly citrus pectin.

In the late 1980s and early 1990s, researchers began to experiment with modified citrus pectin (MCP). This is pectin that's processed to split the complex carbohydrates into smaller sugar units that can be absorbed into the bloodstream.

MCP is rich in a specific sugar molecule called galactose that attaches to break away cancer cells and effectively neutralizes them because, once attached to MCP, the cancer cells lose their ability to clump together and penetrate normal cells. These neutralized cancer cells then circulate until they either die or are destroyed by the immune system.

Also, MCP can attach to tumor cells and help inhibit the cancer from growing and developing into the more advanced stages.

The evidence speaks for itself

So far, most of the cancer research on MCP has been conducted on animals or with cells in the laboratory. The results, however, are impressive. For instance, in one study, colon tumors were implanted in mice. The control group received untreated water. The others received either a low dose of MCP (0.8 mg/mL) or a high dose of MCP (1.6 mg/mL) in their drinking water. When compared to the control group, the low dose resulted in a 38 percent decrease in tumor size, and the high dose treatment resulted in a 70 percent reduction in tumor size.[40]

Some clinical studies on MCP used by cancer patients have been conducted, but only patients with very advanced cancer, for whom all other treatments had failed and no other therapies were available, were allowed to participate. But, even in this "worst case" scenario, over 20 percent experienced an overall clinical benefit along with an improvement in their quality of life. Furthermore, in 24 percent of the cases, the cancer stabilized during the first 8 weeks of treatment and 20 percent remained stabilized over the 16-week period. In 12 percent of the cases, the disease stabilized for longer than 24 weeks while on the MCP.[41]

Special use for biopsies

There's another area where I feel MCP should be used routinely, and that's for biopsies. Biopsies can actually increase the risk of spreading a cancer. When you cut or puncture a tumor, cancerous cells are released into the surrounding tissue where they can be picked up by the bloodstream or lymph system and transported practically anywhere in the body. And while the newer needle biopsies are less invasive, studies have shown there is still an increased risk of spreading the cancer throughout the needle trail. That's why I recommend taking MCP for a week before and 2–4 weeks after a biopsy.

Choosing the dose

In practically all of the cancer studies, a dosage of 15 grams a day was used (5 grams taken three times during the day). This dosage for cancer is generally used as long as the cancer is active or present—even as long as a year. After that period, you can move to a maintenance dose of 3 to 5 grams per day.

For biopsies, I recommend taking 15 grams a day of MCP (5 grams, three times a day) for a week before the procedure and then for 2—4 weeks afterward.

MCP is totally safe. There are no serious side effects, but it's possible that some people might initially experience a little intestinal gas or mild stomach discomfort. This is temporary and not uncommon when increasing the amount of any type of fiber in the diet.

Where to find quality MCP

The studies I've referenced used a product called PectaSol, which is marketed in this country by EcoNugenics. They've also come out with a newer MCP product called PectaSol-C, with improved absorbability. Both are quality products that I highly recommend.

PectaSol and PectaSol-C come in powder form, which can be mixed with water or juice. PectaSol-C is also available in capsules (6 capsules are equivalent to 5 grams of powder). Both products are designed to be taken on an empty stomach, at least one hour before or after food. You can order PectaSol or PectaSol-C directly from EcoNugenics at *econugenics.com* or 1-800-308-5518.

Medicinal mushroom extract

One of the most common complementary cancer therapies—and likely one you've heard of before—is the use of medicinal mushrooms. While many doctors in other countries use extracts of these mushrooms as primary cancer therapies, doctors and other health care practitioners in the United States use them as complementary therapies alongside conventional cancer treatments.

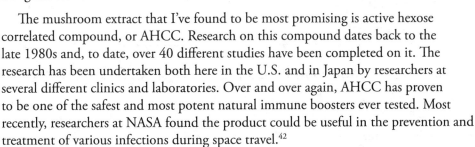

The mushroom extract that I've found to be most promising is active hexose correlated compound, or AHCC. Research on this compound dates back to the late 1980s and, to date, over 40 different studies have been completed on it. The research has been undertaken both here in the U.S. and in Japan by researchers at several different clinics and laboratories. Over and over again, AHCC has proven to be one of the safest and most potent natural immune boosters ever tested. Most recently, researchers at NASA found the product could be useful in the prevention and treatment of various infections during space travel.[42]

How AHCC works

AHCC works to boost your immune system efficiency and effectiveness by several means, but the most powerful way is by increasing the activity of your body's natural killer (NK) cells. NK cells are a form of white blood cells that provide the first line of defense for dealing with any form of invasion to the body, whether it's a virus, bacteria, or cancer cell. I've compared NK cells to elite soldiers who are immediately called upon to seek and destroy dangerous invaders.

Unlike other white blood cells, inadequate numbers of NK cells are rarely a problem. Instead, research now indicates that it's the activity of the cells that generally determines whether you're sick or healthy. As long as the NK cells are active, everything remains under control. If NK cells lose their ability to either recognize or destroy an invader, however, the situation can deteriorate rapidly. In cancer patients, NK cell activity is a key criterion for estimating the chances of survival.

In addition to increasing NK activity as much as 300 percent or more, AHCC also increases the activity of other key immune cells, like T cells and B cells. [43] But that's not all that AHCC does to help in your fight against cancer. AHCC also increases levels of interferon, a potent compound produced by the body that has been shown to inhibit the replication of viruses. And results from an animal study show that AHCC increases the formation of tumor necrosis factors (TNFs), which are a group of proteins that help destroy cancer cells.

AHCC is nontoxic and poses no danger or ill effects from long-term use. It only makes your immune system more effective at targeting cancer cells and pathogens. Regardless of how you decide to treat your cancer, adding AHCC into the mix will increase your chances of being able to recover from the disease and keep it from recurring.

Usage recommendations

For maximum effectiveness during the active phases of your cancer, I recommend taking AHCC at a dose of 3 grams per day. For maintenance during remission phases, I recommend you take 1 gram per day.

Whether you're taking 3 grams or 1, I suggest dividing the daily dosage, taking half of it at breakfast and half at dinnertime.

The AHCC used in much of the research I've mentioned is sold as ImmPower. In this country, ImmPower can be purchased from Harmony Company (*theharmonyco. com* or 1-888-809-1241).

⏵ Your Action Plan if You Have Colorectal Cancer ⏵

No single therapy—either conventional or complementary—is guaranteed to cure cancer, but knowing your options, making informed decisions, and committing your mind, body, and spirit to the task will greatly improve your chances of surviving this life-threatening disease.

Following are the steps I recommend to help you do just that.

1. **Stick with the healthy diet and lifestyle changes** I've outlined throughout this book for strong digestive system health and overall wellness. Pay especially close attention to the recommendations for preventing colorectal cancer.

2. **Work with your doctor to map out a treatment plan that is best for you** and be sure to include one or more of the powerful natural solutions— Avemar, MCP, and AHCC—to not only boost your immune system during the rigors of conventional treatment, but also to help lessen the treatment side effects, improve your comfort and resilience during the course of treatment, and strengthen your body so it can defend against future cancer threats.

3. **Get connected.** Being diagnosed with cancer can leave you frightened and emotionally distraught. Connecting with others who are facing the same challenges can give you insight and support, as well as empower you to ask

the hard questions, consider the best treatment options, and make the optimal choices for your quality care.

One such group that I recommend is On Top of Cancer.org (*ontopofcancer.org*). It's a non-profit organization, with no ties to a particular medical facility, drug company, or treatment group, so their insight and advice is unbiased.

The organization brings together cancer survivors and families, doctors, researchers, and caregivers to give you support, reduce your anxiety and fear, and give you details on a host of important topics, including survivor tips, alternative cancer treatment, finding the best doctor and hospital, cancer clinical trials, legal and financial aid for cancer patients, caregiver support, and cancer advocacy.

❖ ❖ ❖

In Part II of this book, I've addressed the top digestive issues plaguing our population. I hope that you've found the answers you've been searching for as well as the specific tools and techniques you can put to use to get to the root cause of your GI ailment and to build better digestive health and overall wellness.

Many of the conditions I've covered share common symptoms—including heartburn, indigestion, nausea, excessive gas, diarrhea, and constipation. And in the next section of this book, I'll discuss each of these symptoms, with my specific recommendations for ending the suffering that they bring.

Part III

Addressing Distressing Symptoms

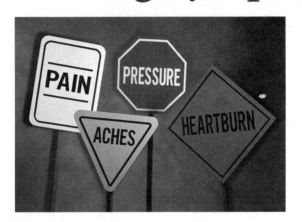

There are several major symptoms of digestive disorders that seem to cause people the most distress, pain, and worry. These are heartburn, indigestion, nausea, excessive gas, diarrhea, and constipation. They are so common, in fact, that I wanted to address them separately, instead of simply discussing them as part of one or more of the most troubling digestive conditions I covered in Part II.

Of course, getting to the root cause of your particular digestive condition should certainly address these troubling symptoms. But, I wanted you to also have a quick and direct way to find relief for symptoms that, while not life-threatening, can certainly be life-altering.

Heartburn

As I mentioned earlier in this book, heartburn is a major symptom of GERD, but not all people with GERD have heartburn and, likewise, not all people with heartburn have GERD. But, with or without other GERD symptoms, chronic heartburn is said to affect at least 60 million Americans, with some estimates as high as 100 million. And some studies suggest that 15 million Americans experience heartburn daily.

Over-the-counter remedies for heartburn crowd pharmacy shelves as well as commercial time slots on television. But, as I explained previously, while some of these drugs provide short-term relief, they don't address the underlying causes of heartburn and may, in fact, worsen the condition.

For example, antacids and H2 blockers are designed to treat and prevent digestive problems such as heartburn by changing the pH balance or acidity of your stomach by either binding with stomach acid or blocking this acid production. This action impairs digestion—especially the digestion of protein, which can lead to nutritional deficiencies as well as digestive problems further down the GI tract, such as excess gas and pain in the colon.

Other drugs for heartburn have proven to be even more dangerous. Take Propulsid (cisapride), for example. This drug, prescribed to treat nighttime heartburn, has been linked with numerous reports of heart rhythm abnormalities and over 100 deaths. In fact, the potential for serious heart problems or even fatality from this drug is so great that Propulsid is no longer being marketed in the U.S.

And an October 2005 article in the *Wall Street Journal* revealed an alarming link between heartburn and esophageal cancer. Research suggests that drugs used to prevent and treat heartburn could be contributing to the rapid rise in the number of cases of this aggressive and deadly type of cancer.

There's simply no reason to endanger your health this way in order to find heartburn relief. As is the case with heartburn and the other common digestive systems that I'll cover in this chapter of the book, there are safe, natural solutions that do more than simply relieve symptoms—they actually heal the digestive tract and promote overall good health. I recommend you take almost the same steps for heartburn as you would for full-blown GERD.

Please turn the page for your action plan for heartburn.

▌▌▌➤ Your Action Plan for Heartburn ▌▌▌➤

1. **Eat a healthy, low-fat diet.** Make a conscious effort to also steer clear of the most common heartburn "trigger foods" such as spicy dishes, fried and high-fat foods, tomatoes and tomato-based products, citrus fruits, garlic, onions, mints, alcoholic beverages, caffeinated coffee and tea, and carbonated drinks. Also, avoid excess salt. Instead, experiment with healthful herbs and spices to enhance the flavor of your food.

   It's also a good idea to eat smaller meals spread throughout the day, to eat slowly and chew thoroughly, and never eat if you're not hungry or if you're upset. After eating, wait at least an hour before exercising, and at least three hours before lying down.

   As a bonus, your healthy eating habits should help you lose excess pounds, which helps reduce the pressure on your abdomen that can cause acid reflux and heartburn.

2. **Drink at least 8–10 eight-ounce glasses of pure, clean water every day.** This helps to keep stray stomach acid from getting into your esophagus, and also promoted good digestion overall. Drink one to two glasses of water when you get up in the morning and a half hour before meals. And take your nutritional supplements at meal times with tall glasses of water.

3. **Stop smoking.** This bad habit has been shown in studies to increase your risk of acid reflux and the heartburn that often results, as well as a host of other health problems.

4. **Avoid tight-fitting clothing** that can constrict your abdomen.

5. **Chew gum.** This simple strategy helps to soothe the esophagus and wash digestive acids back down into the stomach where they belong. Choose a brand sweetened with xylitol, which has been shown to promote dental health and reduce oral bacteria levels.

6. **Try hydrochloric acid.** If you are over 50 years of age, a natural decline in your hydrochloric acid production may be contributing to acid reflux and heartburn, in which case supplementation can help.

   I always recommend betaine hydrochloride, which you can get at health food stores. One really important point to remember is to take one or two tablets after you eat, not before or during your meal. You want your stomach to produce and secrete as much acid as it can before adding the additional acid.

7. **Add digestive enzymes.** In addition to hydrochloric acid, there are dozens of digestive enzymes on the market that can help re-acidify your intestinal tract, improve your overall digestive capabilities, and relieve heartburn symptoms.

A good product will include acids and enzymes similar to those produced by the stomach, like pepsin and betaine hydrochloride. It should also include enzymes commonly produced by the pancreas and those present in the bile from the gallbladder.

If you can't find a good digestive enzyme product at a health food store, call Progressive Laboratories at 1-800-527-9512 or visit their website for more information, *progressivelabs.com*. They sell an excellent product called Digestin #987. Just follow the directions on the bottle.

8. **Take deglycyrrhizinated licorice (DGL).** This herbal extract promotes your gastrointestinal tract's natural defense mechanisms, increases production of protective mucosal cells, and helps reduce inflammation.

   The suggested dose of DGL is two tablets, chewed about 20 minutes before meals, three times a day. Use only chewable DGL—it must be mixed with saliva in order to be effective. Unlike regular licorice, DGL will not cause water retention, raise blood pressure, or lower testosterone levels. This supplement, which is also beneficial for ulcers and canker sores, can be found in most health food stores.

9. **Try D-limonene.** Orange peel extract, and specifically its active ingredient—d-limonene—is another natural solution for heartburn. It floats to the surface of the contents in your stomach and creates a protective lining that helps prevent gastric secretions from sneaking back into your esophagus. It also adds density to your stomach contents, encouraging them to empty properly into your small intestine.

   In a double-blind, placebo-controlled study, 83% of people taking 1,000 mg of d-limonene per day experienced relief of their heartburn pain. You can find d-limonene at health food stores or through a variety of online retailers.

10. **Raise the head of your bed by 4–6 inches.** Make sure you do this by inserting blocks, bricks, or a wedge made specifically for this purpose and available at most medical supply stores, under your mattress...and not by adding pillows under your head. Additional pillows cause your body to bend at the waist near your stomach and can actually aggravate nighttime reflux and heartburn symptoms.

11. **Keep a glass of water by your bed.** If you experience any uncomfortable burning sensations that wake you up, you can take a quick sip to wash stray acids back into your stomach.

To track your success with this Action Plan, I highly recommend that you record the exact steps you're taking to address your heartburn each day, as well as the symptoms you are experiencing at the time, and how you are feeling emotionally.

Putting these details on paper is an excellent way to see what works for you. It's also a great way to document the improvements you're experiencing and just how far you've come using safe, natural solutions to your digestive problem.

Turn to pages 135–136 for sample pages that makes tracking this information simple. Use these pages as your master copy and photocopy more pages to fill in with your details.

Indigestion

Indigestion, also known as dyspepsia, is usually described as a feeling of uncomfortable fullness both during and after a meal, as well as burning or pain in your abdominal area between the lower end of your chest bone and your navel. Indigestion is often a symptom of GERD and peptic ulcers. And nausea and bloating are other symptoms sometimes associated with indigestion.

Stomach upset can be caused by a number of factors, including overeating, eating hard-to-digest or spicy foods, drinking alcoholic beverages, smoking, certain medications, and physical or emotional stress.

? Did You Know...

Chronic indigestion can be a sign of impending heart problems. Indigestion, including abdominal bloating and fullness, as well as other abdominal symptoms such as pain, excessive gas, or nausea, can indicate that your body is struggling to break down fats, proteins, and carbohydrates.

When this happens, blood is shunted to your GI organs to aid digestion, which leaves less blood and oxygen for the heart. This, in turn, makes your heart more vulnerable to ischemia (lack of blood flow) and arrhythmias (irregular heartbeats).

Indigestion can often be addressed effectively with some commonsense dietary and lifestyle changes. If you give these a try and are still experiencing regular indigestion, there are supplements you can take that often bring relief.

⟫ Your Action Plan for Indigestion ⟫

1. **Eat several small, low-fat meals** throughout the day.

2. **Chew your food well and don't overeat.**

3. **Try not to chew with your mouth open, talk while chewing, or eat too fast.** These habits can cause you to swallow excess air, which aggravates indigestion.

4. **Build more raw fruits and vegetables into your diet.** They contain vital organic elements, particularly enzymes that help digest proteins, fats, carbohydrates, and soluble fiber.

5. **Eat cultured or fermented foods**, such as sauerkraut, tofu, tamari, and miso, on a regular basis.

6. **Avoid foods that are known contributors to stomach upset**, including chocolate, fats, milk, orange juice, spicy and fried foods, sugar, and tomato products.

7. **Avoid coffee, carbonated beverages, and alcohol.** These are all well-known stomach lining irritants.

8. **Never eat when you're emotionally upset or not hungry.**

9. **Drink at least 8-10 eight ounce glasses of pure, clean water each day.** But try to drink fluids after meals, rather than during them.

10. **Soothe your stomach with ginger tea.** For centuries, traditional Chinese medicine has valued ginger as a tonic for digestion. It's commonly used for indigestion today because it absorbs and neutralizes toxins in the stomach. It also eases the transport of substances through the digestive tract and decreases irritation to intestinal walls. Ginger tea is available in health food stores. Similarly, you can try chamomile or peppermint tea, which are also known to have a relaxing effect and to relieve indigestion, heartburn, and flatulence.

11. **Stop smoking.** The virtually endless list of health risks associated with this habit includes stomach irritation.

12. **Limit or stop using medications that are known to irritate the stomach lining**, such as aspirin, NSAIDs, steroid medications, certain antibiotics, thyroid medicines, and even estrogen and oral contraceptives.

13. **Get plenty of rest.** Quality sleep helps keep stress at bay and gives your body time to repair, recharge, and regenerate. This is essential for healthy digestion as well as overall good health.

14. **Find other ways to decrease physical and emotional stress**, such as relaxation therapy or yoga.

If these diet and lifestyle changes aren't enough to stop your indigestion, then consider these next steps...

15. **Take a probiotic supplement** to create balanced bacterial flora in your bowels and improve digestion throughout your gastrointestinal tract.

16. **Add digestive enzymes.** These can help re-acidify your intestinal tract improve your overall digestive capabilities, and help soothe indigestion.

A good product will include acids and enzymes similar to those produced by the stomach, like pepsin and betaine hydrochloride. It should also include enzymes commonly produced by the pancreas and those present in the bile from the gallbladder.

If you can't find a good digestive enzyme product at a health food store, call Progressive Laboratories at 1-800-527-9512 or visit their website for more information, *progressivelabs.com*. They sell an excellent product called Digestin #987. Just follow the directions on the bottle.

17. **Take deglycyrrhizinated licorice (DGL).** This herbal extract promotes your gastrointestinal tract's natural defense mechanisms, increases production of protective mucosal cells, and helps reduce inflammation.

The suggested dose of DGL is two tablets, chewed about 20 minutes before meals, three times a day. Use only chewable DGL—it must be mixed with saliva in order to be effective. Unlike regular licorice, DGL will not cause water retention, raise blood pressure, or lower testosterone levels. This supplement, which is also beneficial for ulcers and canker sores, can be found in most health food stores.

18. **Try herbal bitters.** Bitters activate the bitter-taste receptors on the tongue, which, in turn, stimulate the secretion of digestive juices. Several herbs are considered bitters. They include dandelion root, wormwood, chamomile flowers, goldenseal, and gentian root.

Gentian root is probably the most used since it contains one of the most bitter substances known to man (a glycoside called amarogentin). European studies have shown that gentian products can effectively relieve indigestion. In this country gentian is available in powder form, capsules, or as a concentrated extract. For digestive purposes the extracts seem to be more effective and convenient. These are available at most health food stores and from a variety of online retailers.

Generally a couple of drops in a little water taken about 15 to 20 minutes before meals will help with indigestion. (Be aware that too large a dose may cause vomiting. This stuff is bitter!)

· · · · · · · · · · · · · · · · · · ·*Track Your Success!*· · · · · · · · · · · · · · · · · · · ·

To track your success with this Action Plan, I highly recommend that you record the exact steps you're taking to address your indigestion each day, as well as the symptoms you are experiencing at the time, and how you are feeling emotionally.

Putting these details on paper is an excellent way to see what works for you. It's also a great way to document the improvements you're experiencing and just how far you've come using safe, natural solutions to your digestive problem.

Turn to pages 135–136 for sample pages that makes tracking this information simple. Use these pages as your master copy and photocopy more pages to fill in with your details.

Nausea

Nausea is the sensation of unease in the stomach, usually paired with the urge to vomit. It often emanates from organs of the upper gastrointestinal tract, including the esophagus, stomach, and small intestine; as well as from organs peripheral to the digestive system, such as the liver, pancreas, and gallbladder.

Motion sickness and vertigo are particular kinds of nausea that result from disequilibrium. Nausea can also result from medications, such as chemotherapy regimens and anesthesia. When related to pregnancy, nausea is known as "morning sickness," even though women can suffer with this condition during all hours of the day and night. It's estimated that 80 percent of pregnant women experience some degree of nausea during their first trimester due to wide hormonal fluctuations.

Although nausea can be miserable, it's generally not a serious medical condition.

Ⅲ➡ Your Action Plan for Nausea Ⅲ➡

1. **Start with controlled breathing.** Several studies involving subjects who had just undergone surgery and were feeling nauseated found that a slow, deep breathing technique helped to significantly reduce nausea. When you're feeling a bout of nausea, try to inhale slowly through your nose and exhale slowly through your mouth for two to five minutes.

2. **Take ginger root.** Ginger has been used by Indian women as a morning sickness remedy for centuries. And in recent years, ginger's effectiveness against nausea and motion sickness has been well documented. In fact, in several studies, ginger was demonstrated to be far superior to Dramamine, the popular over-the-counter anti-nausea preparation. And it works directly on the gastrointestinal tract, rather than through the central nervous system, as most anti-nausea drugs do.

   Ginger root products can vary widely in quality and potency, so it's important to use ginger supplements from a reputable provider. The gingerroot that I use comes from Penn Herb Company, Ltd. (*pennherb.com* or 1-800-523-9971). For nausea, the generally recommended dosage is 500–600 mg every three to four hours.

3. **Try Sea-Band wristlets.** One way to address nausea—whether from gastrointestinal upset or other causes—is stimulate the acupuncture point P6 (Nei Kuan). This point is about 2 inches above the inside of your wrist. Now there's a product called Sea-Band that takes advantage of this "anti-nausea" acupuncture point.

   Sea-Band is a pair of 1" wide woven-elasticized bands with a plastic ball-shaped button sewn inside. A band is worn around each wrist so that the button places constant pressure on the P6 acupuncture point. The product, which closely resembles a tennis-type sweatband, has reportedly been used successfully to treat motion sickness on ships, morning sickness, and the nausea often associated with chemotherapy.

Sea-Band sells for about $10 and is widely available from online retailers and pharmacies. However, there's no reason you can't make your own using a needle and thread, a small round ball-shaped button, and two tennis wrist sweatbands.

If you don't want to make the anti-nausea bands, or happen to leave them at home, you can always massage the P6 point on both wrists for three to five minutes, as often as needed.

• *Track Your Success!* •

To track your success with this Action Plan, I highly recommend that you record the exact steps you're taking to address your nausea each day, as well as the symptoms you are experiencing at the time, and how you are feeling emotionally.

Putting these details on paper is an excellent way to see what works for you. It's also a great way to document the improvements you're experiencing and just how far you've come using safe, natural solutions to your digestive problem.

Turn to pages 135–136 for sample pages that makes tracking this information simple. Use these pages as your master copy and photocopy more pages to fill in with your details.

Excessive Gas

Although we don't like to talk about it, everybody passes gas. In fact, most people have more than 20 gas-passing "episodes" each day, releasing up to four pints of gas in the process. But just because it's normal doesn't mean it's pleasant. Excessive gas can result in bloating and discomfort. And the belching and flatulence it causes can be embarrassing.

The details on gas

The gas in your body is made up of a number of different vapors, including oxygen and nitrogen from the air we breathe and swallow, as well as carbon dioxide, hydrogen, and methane, which result from digestive processes throughout your GI tract.

? Did You Know...

Only about a third of the population produces methane gas, the most malodorous of all gases from the human digestive tract. Females tend to produce more than males do, and there may be a genetic component to methane gas production, as it seems to be a familial trait.

Much of the foul-smelling gas produced in your digestive system comes from the bacteria in your bowels. Food substances that aren't absorbed in the small intestine and are passed on to the large intestine become fodder for these bacteria. These food substances are primarily sugars and carbohydrates.

Causes of excess gas

Gas can occur as a result of the foods you eat and the way they are (or aren't) digested. Here's a look at some of the most common culprits of food-related gas.

Sugars		
Type	**Food Sources**	**Details**
Raffinose	Beans, cabbage, Brussels sprouts, broccoli, asparagus, other vegetables, whole grains	Beans contain the largest amount of this complex sugar.
Lactose	Milk and milk products, such as cheese and ice cream; processed foods, such as bread, cereal, and salad dressings	Many people have low levels of lactase, the enzyme needed to digest lactose. Lactose intolerance is common in Africans, Native Americans, and Asians. Also, as people age, their production of natural digestive enzymes decreases, resulting in gas from lactose-containing foods.
Fructose	Artichokes, pears, onions, and wheat	Also used as a sweetener in sodas and fruit drinks.
Sorbitol	Apples, peaches, pears, and prunes — Dietetic foods and sugar-free candies and gums	This is a natural sugar found in some fruits, but it's also used as an artificial sweetener in many diet foods. It is particularly well known for causing gas.

(Continued on next page...)

Fiber		
Type	**Food Sources**	**Details**
Soluble	Oat bran, beans, peas, and most fruits	Soluble fiber dissolves in water and creates a soft, lubricating gel in the intestines. It isn't digested until it reaches the colon, where it can cause gas.
Insoluble	Wheat bran and some vegetables	This fiber passes through the intestines undigested and produces little gas.
Starches		
	Potatoes, corn, pasta, wheat	Starches produce gas when they're broken down in the large intestine.
Beverages		
	Carbonated drinks, beer, wine, fruit drinks	Although not true "foods," beverages are elements of your diet that can cause gas, too.

? Did You Know...

Contrary to conventional wisdom, coffee with your meal can help reduce gas rather than add to your digestive woes. Coffee stimulates stomach acid, which helps improve digestion and reduce gas production. Just remember to drink it in moderation.

Another cause for excessive gas is swallowing too much air. This can happen when you drink through a straw, eat or drink too fast, suck on candy, chew gum with your mouth open, or swallow often when you're nervous. It can also be caused by smoking, chewing tobacco, or eating with dentures that don't fit properly. This type of excess gas is often released through belching or burping, but can also lead to flatulence.

Medicines and medical conditions

Excessive gas can come from other sources, including a number of medicines and medical conditions. For instance, antibiotics, NSAIDs, certain diabetes drugs, and

---

A Surprising Cause of Chronic Bad Breath

If you're troubled by chronic bad breath and have checked your teeth, gums, throat, and sinuses for problems, but turned up empty-handed...and if brushing, gargling, eating breath mints, and chewing gum don't help, you may have to look down lower for the answer to your problem.

As the bacteria in your colon breaks down undigested food and produces certain gases, some of the gases are absorbed into your blood and exhaled through your lungs. In fact, as much as 20 percent of the hydrogen produced in the colon is exhaled in your breath. So if your digestive system is not working properly, your breath may be foul-smelling.

The best solution for this bad breath problem is to nourish or replenish the good bacteria in your gut.

Drug chart: excessive gas		
Drug Type—Prokinetic agents		
Brand Name	**Generic Name**	**Potential Side Effects**
Reglan	metoclopramide	Diarrhea; less frequently, may cause involuntary movement of limbs, restlessness, drowsiness, muscle tremor, spasms, breast discharge
Drug Type—Other Agents		
Brand Name	**Generic Name**	**Potential Side Effects**
Actidose-Aqua, CharcoCaps	activated charcoal	Black stools, abdominal pain
Beano	alpha-galactosidase	No known side effects
Pepto-Bismol	bismuth subsalicylate	Dark tongue, grayish-black stools; excessive doses may cause anxiety, constipation, dizziness
Lactaid	lactase	No known side effects
Xifaxan	rifaximin	Headache, constipation, hives and itchiness
Gas Relief, Gas-X, Mylanta Gas, Phazyme	simethicone	No known side effects
Source: Adapted from, Harvard Medical School, *The Sensitive Gut Report* (Boston: Harvard Health Publications, 2010)		

cholesterol-lowering drugs have all been known to increase gas production. This is probably because these medications tend to disrupt the normal chemistry of the digestive system. Also, drugs encapsulated with a sorbitol filler can cause gas because the sorbitol is difficult to digest.

As you know from reading about specific digestive health conditions in Part II of this book, there are digestive ailments that are associated with excess gas, including colitis, Crohn's disease, IBS, ulcers, lactose intolerance, and celiac disease. These conditions interfere with normal, healthy digestion, and excess gas is often a result.

Also, people who have had major surgery on digestive system organs, including colon cancer resection, colon reconstruction, gastric bypass, and gall bladder removal, may also experience an increase in gas after the procedure.

Gas pain

Surprisingly, gas volume and gas pain don't necessarily go hand in hand. People who suffer with gas pain usually have about the same amount of gas that others do, but it affects them more intensely. For instance, people with IBS often have symptoms of gas pain, and research indicates that they also have more sensitive bowels than average.

Some people with gas pain and bloating have bowels with sluggish peristalsis, meaning the muscular contractions of the intestines aren't sufficient to push matter through at a healthy pace. This can cause toxins to accumulate in the gut and intestinal gas to back up into the stomach.

There are a number of simple steps you can take to cut down or even eliminate excess gas from your life, and I've listed them in the Action Plan on the next page.

⮕ Your Action Plan for Excessive Gas ⮕

1. **Identify and cut back on foods that trigger your gas.** Not everyone reacts to the same foods the same way, so this may take a bit of detective work. Track the foods you are eating and the gas symptoms you are suffering to make the connection. Focus first on foods I've outlined for you in the chart on pages 108–109, as these are common gas-creating foods.

2. **If you increase the fiber in your diet, do it slowly.** With a low-fiber diet, your body was likely not producing adequate digestive enzymes. This should adjust eventually, as you continue your healthy, high-fiber diet.

3. **While you wait for your body's natural digestive enzyme production to come up to speed, take supplemental digestive enzymes** to help your body better process the foods you eat and reduce chances of excess gas production. (However, as you age, your body's natural production of these enzymes declines, so you may need to continue with the supplements indefinitely.) I recommend the product Digestin #987, made by Progressive Laboratories (*progressivelabs.com* or 1-800-527-9512).

4. **Create a healthy bacterial balance in your bowels with probiotics.** Since plenty of the gas you're suffering from is created by intestinal bacteria, it makes sense to ensure that those bacteria are healthy, balanced, and working toward optimal digestion of the foods you eat. Probiotics will also help to keep your bowels moving properly so that food matter doesn't sit in your intestines too long. This helps prevent your intestinal bacteria from feeding too long and producing excess gas.

5. **Drink before, not during your meals.** When you drink liquids with your meal, it tends to wash away some of the digestive acids in your stomach, leaving your stomach less able to properly digest the food you eat. Drink about a half hour before your meal to prime your digestive acids instead of watering them down.

6. **Eat and drink at a leisurely pace.** Don't rush through meals or gulp down drinks when you're thirsty. This just increases the air you take into your digestive system and promotes gas formation. Eat slowly. Chew thoroughly. And enjoy.

7. **Avoid drinking through a straw or eating with loose dentures.** Both of these can increase the air you take in and produce unwanted gas.

8. **Eliminate habits like smoking and chewing tobacco** that can fill your stomach with air and lead to gas. These are terrible habits for other health reasons anyway.

9. **If you chew gum** (and it's actually recommended for soothing acid reflux), make sure you **chew small pieces with your mouth closed** so you don't swallow excess air.

10. **Consider the medications you take regularly and determine if these might be contributing to your gas problems.** If so, work with your doctor to adjust your dosage or eliminate the drugs entirely.

11. **Try activated charcoal** if you have a bout of bad gas. It attracts and neutralizes gas in the lower intestines and is available in easy-to-take capsules and tablets through a variety of online retailers and in most health food stores. Follow label instructions.

12. **Take peppermint oil**, a proven remedy for relieving gas pain and bloating. I suggest taking only enteric-coated capsules, which don't break down until they've passed through your stomach. The dose used in most studies is one to two capsules containing 0.2 mL of oil twice a day. I also recommend a cup of fragrant peppermint tea after meals to aid digestion. (Even though coffee can improve digestion, I prefer tea for its many other health-enhancing benefits.) Look for peppermint oil capsules and tea in your health food store.

13. **Exercise regularly.** Of the many health benefits you'll get from regular exercise, improved digestion is one of the most important. Exercise actually massages your internal organs, keeps your digestion moving along, and prevents food from stalling, stagnating, and becoming a breeding ground for excess gas.

• • *Track Your Success!* **• •**

To track your success with this Action Plan, I highly recommend that you record the exact steps you're taking to address your excess gas each day, as well as the symptoms you are experiencing at the time, and how you are feeling emotionally.

Putting these details on paper is an excellent way to see what works for you. It's also a great way to document the improvements you're experiencing and just how far you've come using safe, natural solutions to your digestive problem.

Turn to pages 135–136 for sample pages that makes tracking this information simple. Use these pages as your master copy and photocopy more pages to fill in with your details.

Diarrhea

Diarrhea is typically defined as loose, watery stools that come on urgently and frequently—usually defined as more than three times a day. It can also be accompanied by abdominal pain, gas, bloating, and even nausea.

As you learned earlier, when you eat, your stomach secretes large amounts of water to transform the food into a sludgy liquid called chyme. The small intestine, pancreas, and gallbladder also add secretions to keep the food in an easy-to-move liquid state. Then, the lower small intestine and colon absorb the water, turning the undigested food matter into a more solid form. This is your stool or feces.

Abnormal amounts of water in the stool can be the result of your stomach or small intestine secreting too much fluid, the lower small intestine and colon absorbing too little liquid, or the chyme passing too quickly through the small intestine and colon, and not allowing for proper water absorption by these organs.

There are two types of diarrhea—chronic and acute, and they each have different causes and recommended treatments.

Chronic diarrhea

Chronic diarrhea is often related to functional GI disorders, such as IBS, IBD, and colon cancer, or immune deficiency diseases, such as AIDS. This type of diarrhea is often accompanied by other symptoms, such as blood or mucus in the stool and weight loss. And with IBS, diarrhea and constipation are alternating symptoms.

The key to resolving chronic diarrhea is to address the underlying condition. This book has covered a wide variety of solutions for digestive conditions that have chronic diarrhea as a symptom.

Acute diarrhea

Acute diarrhea is quite common. In fact, most adults have bouts of it several times a year. But it usually only lasts a few days and doesn't lead to any serious complications.

Drug chart: diarrhea		
Drug Type—Antidiarrheal agents		
Brand Name	**Generic Name**	**Potential Side Effects**
Lomotil, Logen	diphenoxylate, atropine	Abdominal discomfort, constipation. Less frequently, may cause blurred vision, urinary discomfort, dry mouth or skin, rapid heartbeat, restlessness, or warm, flushed skin.
Imodium, Imodium A-D	loperamide	Abdominal discomfort, constipation. Less frequently, may cause drowsiness, dizziness, dry mouth, nausea, vomiting, rash.
Source: Adapted from, Harvard Medical School, *The Sensitive Gut Report* (Boston: Harvard Health Publications, 2010)		

This type of diarrhea is usually brought on by a bacterial, viral, or parasitic infection. It can also be caused by an adverse reaction to medication or food intolerance. Here's a breakdown of some of the more common causes of acute diarrhea:

Type	Specific Pathogen/Cause	Details
Viral	Rhinovirus, rotavirus, norovirus, influenza	These viruses cause viral gastroenteritis, an infection of the stomach and small intestines, and are the most common cause of diarrhea worldwide.
Bacterial	*Escherichia coli, Shigella, Vibrio cholerae, Clostridium difficile*	Produce toxins that cause diarrhea.
	Salmonella, Campylobacter, Staphylococcus aureus, Clostridium perfringens	Food poisoning is caused by these bacteria, which produce toxins in food before or after it's eaten.
Parasitic	*Giardia, Cryptosporidium*, roundworms, tapeworms	Parasitic infections are not common causes of diarrhea in the U.S., and are usually picked up by drinking untreated water when traveling abroad, or drinking lake or river water when camping or hiking.
Drug-related	Antacids, supplements containing magnesium, antibiotics, NSAIDs, medications to control irregular heartbeat, chemotherapy medications, high blood pressure medications	This type of diarrhea usually begins soon after starting on the drug.

? **Did You Know...**

Antibiotics kill the natural balance of bacteria in the gut and can make it more vulnerable to a particularly toxic bacterium known as *Clostridium difficile*. This pathogen is commonly acquired in hospitals, but is now showing up in individuals who have neither been on antibiotics nor been in the hospital, which indicates it is becoming more virulent.

Complications

Acute diarrhea is your body's attempt to clear an unwanted element from the intestines. In most cases, it's best to let your body do this cleansing work on its own, while making sure that you keep sufficiently hydrated to make up for the fluid loss that takes place.

This is important, because dehydration is the most common complication of diarrhea. It often occurs in adults with acute diarrhea who also have nausea and vomiting, making it difficult to keep down any liquids. And it can be quite serious in children because they tend to become dehydrated quite quickly. In fact, diarrhea is the second leading cause of death worldwide in children under the age of five.[44]

Signs of dehydration include dry lips and mouth, eyes that look dull or sunken, scant and concentrated urine, and lethargy. Severe dehydration can cause fainting, weakness, confusion, an accumulation of acid in the blood, and even kidney failure, shock, and coma.

For mild cases of diarrhea, stay hydrated with water and other clear liquids, like broth, and ginger ale. No sugar-added apple juice is also a good alternative, but stay away from citrus drinks. Coffee and alcohol are also no-no's because they're dehydrating. You should also avoid lactose-containing foods, like most dairy products, because they can exacerbate diarrhea.

When diarrhea is chronic or severe, it can lead to an electrolyte imbalance. Most often, it will result in sodium and potassium deficiencies. Hydrating with electrolyte-replacement drinks is advisable in this case. I like HEED sports drinks by Hammer Nutrition. As I mentioned earlier in this book, they are formulated for endurance athletes and are made from complex carbohydrates, sweetened with stevia and xylitol, provide a full spectrum of all-chelated minerals, and they come in a variety of flavors. They can be purchased at numerous running, cycling, multi-sport, and outdoor outfitter stores. Go online to *hammernutrition.com* to find a dealer near you, or you can order directly from this site.

Other options are oral rehydration solutions (ORS), which are liquids made specifically for rehydration purposes, and include Rehydralyte for adults and Pedialyte and Infalyte for children and infants.

If this still isn't enough to rehydrate you, seek help from your doctor. You may have to receive fluids and nutrients by IV to counter what you've lost.

After rehydrating, you should resume eating solid foods when any accompanying nausea and vomiting subsides. Start with easy-to-manage choices, like apple sauce, bananas, cereal, rice, potatoes, and lactose-free items. You can expand on this once your diarrhea subsides and you regain your appetite.

Traditional treatments

Conventional medicine offers a number of medicines to counteract diarrhea. Some, called absorbents, bind with water in the small intestines and colon to make stools less watery, others, referred to as anti-motility medications, relax the muscles of the small intestines and colon and slow the flow of intestinal contents. And bimuth-containing compounds, such as Pepto-Bismol, are thought to have antibiotic-like properties which affect bacteria that can cause diarrhea, and also anti-inflammatory properties that can lead to reduced water secretion by the intestines.

Here's a look at some of the most common diarrhea medicines.

Type	Common Brands	Details
Absorbents with Attapulgite	Diasorb, Donnagel, Kaopectate Advanced Formula, Parepectolin, Rheaban	Absorbents bind with water in the small intestine to make stools less watery. They can also bind with medications and impair their absorption, so these medications should not be taken at the same time.
Absorbents with Polycarbophil	Konsyl Fiber, Mitrolan, Polycarb	
Anti-Motility Medications	Imodium (loperamide), Lomotil (diphenoxylate)	Imodium is non-prescription and Lomotil is prescription-only. Anti-motility drugs should NOT be used to treat diarrhea related to UC, *Clostridium difficile*, or intestinal bacterial infections as they can lead to increased inflammation and prolonged infection. Also not recommended for children under age 2. If acute diarrhea doesn't improve after 72 hours on an anti-motility drug, discontinue and consult your doctor.
Bismuth-containing Compounds	Pepto-Bismol	Contains bismuth and salicylate (aspirin). Helps reduce inflammation, which may reduce water secretion in the intestines. May turn stool and tongue black. Should not be taken by those with allergies to aspirin or used with other aspirin-containing medications. Can interact with anticoagulants, like warfarin (Coumadin) and lead to excessive bleeding. Can aggravate peptic ulcers. Should not be given to children with influenza or chickenpox, as it may cause Reye's syndrome. Not recommended for children under age 2.

Alternatives to consider for treating diarrhea

As you can plainly see from the chart above, the most common medications for diarrhea come with their own side effects and causes for worry. I especially have concerns about the anti-motility medications, like Imodium and the more powerful Lomotil. This is because, while they may stop your diarrhea, they also bring your body's natural cleansing process to an abrupt halt. This, in turn, can cause a prolonged toxicity problem throughout your body.

There are safe, natural alternatives for treating your diarrhea. Following are the four that I've found most useful.

Enemas

One of the quickest ways to resolve acute diarrhea is with a series of enemas. Although this may seem counter-intuitive at first, it really makes good sense. Diarrhea is your body's attempt to clear out an irritant, and the enemas simply speed this process along.

I recommend flushing the colon with a solution of roughly one quart of distilled water plus one half cup of apple cider vinegar to rid the colon of bacteria or other offending pathogens. This, in turn, should stop your diarrhea.

Lactic Acid Yeast Wafers

If your diarrhea is a result of an imbalance in intestinal bacteria—as is often the case with diarrhea that comes when taking antibiotics—you should immediately start taking Lactic Acid Yeast wafers.

This product quickly restores the natural bacteria in your lower bowel. Usually, chewing two wafers with each meal will do the trick within a day. For small children, one or even ½ of a wafer can be crushed and consumed with food or drink. Lactic Acid Yeast wafers can be purchased through your health care professional, or from Standard Process, (*standardprocess.com* or 1-800-558-8740).

Clay

Since most people still equate clay with dirt and mud, the thought of ingesting clay internally may seem a little unsettling. It shouldn't be. For centuries, various clays have proven very effective at safely stopping diarrhea. In fact, it's been used effectively in China, Germany, and France to effectively treat cholera and to combat dysentery and other forms of diarrhea.

One study from the 1960s involved 35 different individuals whose diarrhea problems were being caused by food poisoning, food allergies, viral infection, spastic colitis, or mucus colitis. Two tablespoons of smectite clay (montmorillonite) were given with distilled water three times a day. (In the food allergy cases, six tablespoons of clay per day were used.) In 34 of the 35 individuals, the diarrhea stopped in an average of 3.8 days. The food allergy–induced diarrhea proved to be the most difficult to resolve, whereas diarrhea from viral infections was the easiest.[46]

Clay 101

Clay is an extremely effective detoxification agent because it possesses the properties of both adsorption and absorption. Adsorption (with a "d") is the process in which substances are drawn to, and stick to, the outside of the clay particles. The outside surface of clay has a negative electrical charge. Toxins and impurities typically carry a positive charge. When the two are in close proximity, they attract and chemically bind together.

Clay also has strong absorption (with a "b") properties. This is where substances are drawn into and become attached to the internal structure of the clay rather than just attaching to the surface area…more in keeping with the way a sponge works.

Also, clay has a uniquely large surface area. This is particularly true of the montmorillonite type of clay, which is structured somewhat like a credit card. The flat surface is negatively charged, with positive charges along the edges. Mineralogists have found that a single gram of this clay has a surface area of 800 square meters. This provides the clay with enormous binding capability when it comes to removing toxins.

By helping to remove toxins and pathogens in your intestines, clay can get to the root of your diarrhea to stop it dead in its tracks.

Additional benefits of clay

One of the benefits of consuming clay orally, in addition to its detoxifying effects, is the wide range of trace minerals you receive. If you look at an analysis of many "consumable" clays, the number of trace minerals present is astounding. Practically every mineral you can imagine will be there—including micro-trace amounts of some known to be toxic, such as lead, arsenic, and cadmium. This has led many people to condemn the consumption of clay.

What is often overlooked, however, is the fact that various other competing minerals in these clays are present in much larger quantities. For example, zinc and copper compete with cadmium, and, when present in sufficient amounts, block cadmium's absorption. This is true of other toxins as well. Clays with the right mineral content have been consumed safely for thousands of years. The key is to only use clays that are known to be safe.

How to use clay to stop diarrhea

Clay powder can be simply mixed with juice or water. Make sure the water is either spring water or distilled if possible. Some people like to mix the powder with water, roll it into small balls, and let them dry in the sunlight. These "pills" can be flavored or left natural, and then sucked on throughout the day, like candy.

When you mix clay, stay away from metal utensils or mixing containers because these can react with the clay. Instead, always use wooden utensils and glass, clay, or ceramic containers.

Typical daily supplemental doses of clay are:

- Infants: ¼ to ½ teaspoon
- Children and small adults: 1 teaspoon
- Adults of medium build: 1 heaping teaspoon
- Adults of large build: 1 tablespoon
- Adults of extra-large build: 1 heaping tablespoon

Since clay has such strong absorptive and adsorptive properties, it is best not to take it with your vitamins or at the same time you take prescription medications, as it may bind to and prevent the action of these. I suggest taking clay on an empty stomach and then waiting at least 4 hours before taking any medications or supplements.

Also, I don't recommend ingesting clay if you have an intolerance to iron or high blood pressure.

Where to get quality clay

One source for clay that I've used for years and can highly recommend is Pascalite, Inc., (*pascalite.com* or 307-347-3872), This is a family operation out of Wyoming. The family actually does the mining of the clay themselves and the clay is a calcium bentonite/montmorillonite type.

Pascalite is a small but efficient operation so please be patient if you call and the phone is busy. You won't find friendlier, more caring individuals. I should also mention that there are some companies on the Internet now falsely claiming to sell Pascalite clay at discount prices. I don't know what you'll get if you order from these companies, but it won't be Pascalite. You won't have that problem if you order directly from the company.

Ileocecal valve adjustment

Your ileocecal valve is a small control device located between your small and large intestines. This little valve has two very important jobs to do. First, it blocks toxic contents in the large intestine from backing up into the small intestine. Second, it keeps food products in the small intestine from passing into the large intestine before they are properly digested.

Unfortunately, your ileocecal valve can sometimes get stuck shut or stuck open. When it's stuck shut, it can lead to constipation and when it's stuck open, it can lead to diarrhea.

When the valve sticks open

When your ileocecal valve is stuck open, the food in your small intestines moves too rapidly into your large intestines and doesn't allow the small intestines enough time to absorb water. Also, waste products from the large intestine can back up into the small intestine, where they are reabsorbed into your body.

Why the valve sticks

There are several reasons why the valve doesn't always work right, but I'll only mention a few of the more common ones here. Sometimes spicy or roughage-type foods will irritate the valve and cause it to stick. Another factor that greatly influences the valve is stress or emotional trauma. Also, people who have had their appendix removed, seem to have more problems with their ileocecal valve. Some researchers believe that the appendix, which is located right next to this valve, acts like "an overflow bag for toxins," holding them until the body can slowly eliminate them without interfering in the workings of the ileocecal valve. So, without an appendix, this safety measure is no longer in place to protect your ileocecal valve.

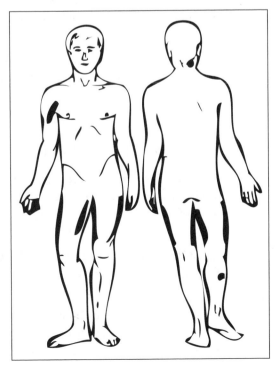

What to do

If your ileocecal valve is stuck open, you can do three things to encourage it to close. The first is to rub specific pressure points on your body associated with ileocecal function. These areas are marked in the illustration to the right. Massage these points with firm pressure for about 10–20 seconds each. No more, no less. You can do this with a vibrator, too, if you find that helpful. Sometimes these pressure points can be quite sore—especially if the valve has been stuck for a long time. But, in general, this simple, noninvasive procedure can instantly correct your valve problem and bring instant relief from your diarrhea.

If you find the pressure point method doesn't work for you, however, there are two more things you can try. One is to manually hold the valve shut for several minutes. To do this, simply place your hand over the valve (it's located about halfway between your belly button and your right hip bone) and push in while at the same time pulling up toward your left shoulder.

Finally, you can try using a cold pack to encourage the ileocecal valve to close. Just place the pack, made of cold water or ice, over the valve for about 15 to 20 minutes.

IIII▶ Your Action Plan for Diarrhea IIII▶

1. **If you have chronic diarrhea associated with an underlying digestive condition, follow the steps outlined in this book to address that condition.** When you tackle root causes this way, you should get relief from associated symptoms, like diarrhea.

2. **If you think your chronic diarrhea is related a food intolerance, keep a journal of the foods you eat and the digestive symptoms that follow.** This way, you'll know which foods to avoid in the future.

3. **If your diarrhea is acute, and not related to an underlying digestive condition, take heart that it will likely resolve on its own in a matter of days.**

4. **Get some soothing medicated wipes.** This will help you clean up without irritating your rectal area, which is a common complication with diarrhea.

5. **Stay hydrated** throughout the course of your diarrhea episode. Drink plenty of water and other clear liquids, like broth, ginger ale, or an electrolyte-replacement drink.

6. **If your diarrhea is severe, try one or more of the four natural therapies** outlined above to help bring it quickly under control. These include enemas, Lactic Acid Yeast wafers, clay, and ileocecal valve adjustment.

7. **Keep your diet basic** while your body works to normalize your bowel movements. Start with easy-to-manage choices, like apple sauce, bananas, cereal, rice, potatoes, and lactose-free items. You can expand on this once your diarrhea subsides and you regain your appetite.

8. **Know when to contact your doctor.** While most cases of diarrhea are mild, there are times when you need to be seen by a medical expert. These are when:

   - You have a fever greater than 101° F

   - You're experiencing moderate or severe abdominal pain

   - You have bloody diarrhea, which could mean severe intestinal inflammation

   - Your diarrhea doesn't improve within 72 hours

   - You can't keep down fluids and become dehydrated

   - You become lethargic, weak, faint, or confused

   - Your diarrhea started after a course of antibiotics. This could indicate an infection by the virulent *Clostridium difficile* bacterium

• **Track Your Success!** •

To track your success with this Action Plan, I suggest that you record the exact steps you're taking to address your diarrhea when it strikes, as well as the symptoms you are experiencing at the time, and how you are feeling emotionally.

Putting these details on paper is an excellent way to see what works for you. It's also a great way to document the improvements you're experiencing and just how far you've come using safe, natural solutions to your digestive problem.

Turn to pages 135–136 for sample pages that makes tracking this information simple. Use these pages as your master copy and photocopy more pages to fill in with your details.

Constipation

At least four million Americans suffer from constipation, accounting for 2.5 million visits to the doctor each year. Constipation seems to affect women more than men, and adults 65 and older more than any other age group. We spend approximately $725 million annually on laxatives to alleviate the problem. But it doesn't seem to be working, In fact, as you'll learn in a minute, it only makes things worse.

What is constipation?

Constipation is often defined as having a bowel movement fewer than three times a week. But, I simply don't agree. You should be moving your bowels at least once a day, and ideally two or three times daily. After all, you eat three meals a day, and each meal creates its own waste products that need to be eliminated.

When your stools pass through your large intestine too slowly, it gets backed up. The stools sit there too long and your colon continues to absorb water from them. The result is waste matter that's hard, dry, and difficult to pass. That's constipation in a nutshell.

Causes and conditions associated with constipation

In most cases, constipation is the result of a poor diet, an inadequate intake of fluids, and insufficient exercise. Some drugs can cause constipation, including painkillers with codeine, antacids that contain aluminum and calcium, calcium channel blockers, antidepressants, anticonvulsants, antispasmodics, and even the diuretics known as "water pills." Supplements with calcium and iron are constipation-causers, too.

Stress and travel can lead to constipation because they interfere with your normal daily routine. Pregnancy and child birth are well known for causing constipation, which is likely the result of the tremendous physical and hormonal changes that occur during

---

Defining Normal: What Is a Healthy Human Stool?

Of course, everybody's different when it comes to bowel habits. But, I think there's a general misconception about what a healthy human stool actually is.

Even medical schools teach that a normal stool is "well formed" or tubular, like a link of sausage. But, history shows that this just isn't the case. And as you may already know, "well-formed" stool can be difficult to pass.

Two physicians, Hugh Trowell and Denis Burkitt, spent most of their careers in Africa, and took note of the African people's large, moist, unformed stool. It spread out in a circle on the ground like cow droppings. And Africans, with their high-fiber vegetable diet and healthy stools, have little problem with constipation.

If you're eating three meals a day, then ideally you should be having three bowel movements a day to eliminate the waste material from those meals. But, at the very minimum, you should have one healthy bowel movement a day. If you're not, then you're constipated and should take the steps outlined in this chapter to address the condition.

Drug chart: constipation		
Drug Type—Prokinetic agents		
Brand Name	**Generic Name**	**Potential Side Effects**
Reglan	metoclopramide	Diarrhea; less frequently may cause involuntary movement of limbs, restlessness, drowsiness, muscle tremor, spasms, breast discharge
Drug Type—Laxatives		
Brand Name	**Generic Name**	**Potential Side Effects**
Colace, Surfak	docusate	Stomach or intestinal cramps, stomach upset, throat irritation
various	mineral oil	May cause deficiencies of fat-soluble vitamins if used regularly; can cause lung damage if accidentally inhaled
MiraLAX	polyethylene glycol	Upset stomach, bloating, cramping, gas
Correctol, Dulcolax, Fleet, others	bisacodyl	Stomach cramps, upset stomach, diarrhea, stomach and intestinal irritation, faintness, irritation or burning in the rectum (from suppositories)
Fleet, Purge	castor oil	Diarrhea, upset stomach, vomiting, irritation, stomach cramping
Ex-Lax, Fletcher's Castoria, Senokot, others	senna	Diarrhea, upset stomach, vomiting, irritation, stomach cramping, pseudomelanosis coli
Total Amount Spent on Laxatives per Year: $725 Million—Source: AARP		
Source: Adapted from, Harvard Medical School, *The Sensitive Gut Report* (Boston: Harvard Health Publications, 2010)		

these life events. Aging is a life process that regularly leads to constipation. In this case, the constipation is probably a result of slower metabolism, a less active lifestyle, and weakened muscles.

Certain diseases are also associated with constipation, including digestive conditions like IBS, Crohn's disease, colon cancer, and diverticulosis (more on this in a minute); metabolic and endocrine diseases such as diabetes, hyperglycemia, and hypothyroidism; and even neurological disorders, like multiple sclerosis, Parkinson's disease, spinal cord injuries, and stroke.

Diverticulosis—another condition commonly found with constipation and a low-fiber diet

Diverticulosis is a condition in which small sacs called diverticula protrude through areas of weakness in the colon wall. This condition is rare in cultures that eat a high-fiber diet. But in the U.S., where low-fiber, highly processed foods are the norm, about half of all adults between the ages of 60 and 80 have diverticulosis.

Diverticulosis usually produces no symptoms. However, a flare-up of diverticulitis (inflammation of the diverticula) can cause severe lower abdominal pain, cramping, and tenderness. To reduce the risk of an attack, doctors generally advise patients with diverticulosis to avoid eating nuts and especially seeds because it's believed that these foods could lodge in the diverticula, triggering symptoms.

Although there's little research to support this hypothesis, it's wise to forego nuts and seeds during a bout of diverticulitis. You can experiment with these foods when you are asymptomatic because some seed-heavy foods, such as tomatoes and strawberries, have numerous health benefits.

And don't be scared off by flaxseed. Grinding flaxseed in a coffee grinder eliminates any potential for the seeds to become lodged in your diverticula. Adding ¼ cup of ground flaxseed to your diet will promote healthy bowel function and decrease the risk of diverticulitis. As a bonus, it will also help lower cholesterol and protect against cancer.

I recommend buying whole flaxseed and grinding it just before using. You can mix it in water or juice (stir and drink quickly, because it thickens as it sits), or sprinkle it on cereal or salads.

Also, follow all the healthy diet recommendations I've outlined for you in this book. They will go a long way to protect against the formation of diverticula and help prevent diverticulitis flare-ups.

Hemorrhoids—a pain from the strain

When you strain to expel constipated feces, you are putting yourself at risk for another painful condition—hemorrhoids.

It's estimated that anywhere from 50 to 75 percent of the adult population have the problem and studies show that Americans are spending in the neighborhood of 75 to 80 million dollars a year on hemorrhoid creams and salves, even though none of the products get rid of the problem. As common as hemorrhoids are, you might expect that there would be some high-tech solution for them by now. Unfortunately, this isn't the case. Surgeons are still "tying off," injecting, freezing, and burning hemorrhoids, just as they have for years. About the only preventative advice offered to the sufferer involves using a stool softener and staying on a high-fiber diet.

Fortunately, if you understand why and how a hemorrhoid develops, you can see there are things you can do to resolve them.

How a hemorrhoid forms

Very simply put, a hemorrhoid is just a distended or bulged vein. Veins, as a general rule, have small check valves or flaps inside to keep blood from pooling or flowing backward. For some reason, these check valves aren't present in the small veins that drain the anal area. Without the check valves, these veins at the end of the system, so to speak, have to support the weight coming from the column of blood above.

This alone is enough to cause problems, but there's even more bad news. These same veins are designed to be more of a light-duty backup system to handle only excess blood flow to the area. Their light-duty structure many times will fail when subjected to extreme strain—like when you're constipated and trying to move your bowels. As a result, the veins bulge, and the bulge can either pop out from between muscle layers in the rectum or move externally through the anal sphincter muscles.

Once the distended vein gets in these positions, the surrounding muscles keep it from returning to its normal location. Exposed and unprotected, the hemorrhoid gets scraped, bumped or aggravated by everything moving through the rectum. Just its presence in the rectum can create the sensation that a bowel movement is needed or was incomplete. The pain can be excruciating.

Current "treatments" for hemorrhoids

The current type of surgical treatment used for hemorrhoids includes rubber band ligation, injection with chemicals to kill exposed tissue, freezing, burning, or surgical removal. Unfortunately, all treatments are uncomfortable to say the least.

A better way

Fortunately, there is another way. To correct hemorrhoids naturally, you have to dilate, stretch and/or slightly separate these muscle bundles to allow the veins to reposition themselves. I have had many patients do this procedure successfully on their own, but I don't recommend it. It shouldn't be difficult to find a doctor to help you with this procedure and it's best to make sure you're dealing only with hemorrhoids before doing anything.

The procedure is quite simple, although not too comfortable. Using a surgical glove and some type of lubricant, one finger is inserted into the rectum and the sphincter muscle is stretched in a circular motion. Then two fingers are inserted, again using a slow, steady, circular stretching motion. Then the procedure is continued with three and then four fingers.

Fortunately, if done properly, one time of this may be all that's needed. Occasionally, it must be performed a couple of times, but not on the same day. This simple procedure can reduce the amount of hemorrhoids protruding from the anus.

You should follow up this procedure with a few more steps to lessen abdominal pressure or abdominal blood pooling to further correct hemorrhoids or prevent new ones from forming.

- Take sitz baths followed by an application of witch hazel for temporary pain relief.

- Follow the action plan at the end of this chapter for eliminating constipation.

- Drink ¼–½ cup of aloe vera gel daily to speed healing in the rectal and anal regions.

- Take a bioflavanoid complex (1,000–4,000 mg daily) along with vitamin C (500–1,000 mg daily) to reduce the pain and bleeding of hemorrhoids, and to strengthen the small blood vessels in the anal area.

- Avoid straining to pass stools.

- Use your leg muscles when you lift. Using the muscles of the stomach and back exerts pressure in the anal region.

- Don't hold your breath when you lift or defecate. This further compresses the abdomen.

- Exercise by walking to strengthen your buttocks and rectal area, which is essential for clearing up hemorrhoids.

- Lose excess weight, especially in the abdominal area, which can add to the type of strain that leads to hemorrhoids.

Misguided bowel habits

As our lives become ever more stressful and hurried, many people simply ignore their body's urge to have a bowel movement. Kids do this because they're too busy playing. Adults have other reasons. Maybe they're in an important meeting, in the car running errands, or somewhere unfamiliar with bathrooms that are unappealing. Whatever the reason, they suppress the urge to purge. And, over time, this leads to constipation.

Another misguided bowel habit that can lead to constipation is, ironically, overuse of laxatives. Often, people start taking laxatives to increase their number of bowel movements and then find they have to take more and more laxatives to continue having bowel movements. Laxatives become a habit or a crutch, leaving the body unable to perform normal bowel elimination on its own.

Get things moving

The most important thing you can do to address your constipation problem is to increase your intake of fiber-rich plant foods. Fresh vegetables, fruits, beans, and grains should make up the majority of your diet, as the fiber in these foods increases both the frequency and quantity of bowel movements. You should also make sure to drink plenty of water and get some exercise most days of the week.

These basic lifestyle changes should be enough to produce regular, healthy bowel movements without the need for laxatives. But, if you find the occasional need to help your bowels along, I suggest using an herbal laxative.

PART III

Is Your Ileocecal Valve Stuck Shut?

In the last chapter, I discussed the ileocecal valve —a small control device located between your small and large intestines—and how it can become stuck open, leading to diarrhea. But this valve can also get stuck shut, which contributes to constipation.

When the valve is stuck in a shut position, your feces cannot be expelled properly from your small intestine into your large intestine. The toxic material backs up and you become constipated. But that's not all. As the fecal matter sits, your small intestine continues to absorb water and toxins back into your body, which puts added pressure on your immune system as well as your digestive system.

To release the value and restore its normal functioning, follow the steps I outlined for you on pages 120–121.

Herbal laxatives

Various herbs work in different methods to stimulate the colon. Some, such as cascara sagrada, induce peristalsis, the normal wave-like motion that pushes stool through the large intestine. This is the same type of motion that helps push your chewed food down your esophagus. Other herbs, such as rhubarb, help draw water into the intestine, which promotes the muscular contractions that promote bowel movements.

Another plant product is actually a combination of three herbs—amla, beleric myrobalan, and *Terminalia chebula*—known as triphala. This formula is the most popular Ayurvedic herbal remedy, and with good reason. I've recommended it in the past for vision support, and there's also evidence that it promotes cardiovascular health. Triphala absorbs liquids into the stool, making it softer and easier to pass. Moister stool is also bulkier, and the increased volume acts as its own stimulant to elimination.

These herbal laxatives are available through a variety of online retailers and in most health food stores. I recommend an herbal laxative that contains cascara sagrada and rhubarb, from Thorne Research (*www.thorne.com* or 1-800-228-1966).

But, before you take any of them, there are a few things I want to point out:

- Herbal laxatives tend to produce initial results within six to eight hours. You don't want to take one then head out to the airport for a long plane ride. A better solution might be to take it at night, so you'll be ready to go just about the time you get up the next morning.

- When you take a laxative, or increase the fiber in your diet significantly, it's imperative to increase your water intake. This will help the fiber do its work effectively.

- No matter what, you shouldn't take any laxative product for more than two weeks. It can lead to the dependence on laxatives that I mentioned earlier.

- If you have or develop diarrhea or loose stools, or any type of abdominal pain, when taking a laxative, stop taking it immediately.

? Did You Know…

Sorbitol is a very common sweetener for sugar-free gums and mints. And it's a natural laxative. Chewing 1–2 pieces of gum with sorbitol is equal to eating a prune!

Keep things moving

Once your intestines have regained their proper muscular motion, and you've begun giving them the proper materials to work with, they shouldn't need any more stimulation. What they do need, however, is something to act on. And that something is fiber.

I've already discussed the importance of fiber in Part I of this book, but let me repeat a few facts here. We should eat 25–30 grams of fiber daily, soluble and insoluble combined, to keep our bowels in good condition. But most Americans consume only about 12–17 grams per day. You may think 30 grams of fiber a day is a high goal, but there are many civilizations in which people eat a plant-based diet and routinely get more than 50 grams of fiber a day.

Aim to increase your daily fiber intake, and make at least 25 percent of your dietary fiber the soluble form. This type of fiber swells up and forms a gel when mixed with water, creating bulk in your stool and acting as a lubricant to help your stools pass easily. Good sources of soluble fiber are fruits, oats, nuts, flaxseed and other seeds, and chia.

Fiber supplements

If you find that you're having difficulty getting enough fiber in your diet on a regular basis, then you may want to add a fiber supplement. In fact, I believe that you absolutely should add a fiber supplement while you're taking a laxative. If you're stimulating your bowel, but there's nothing to push against, you'll just be wasting your time and energy.

A good fiber supplement should contain primarily sources of soluble fiber, including fruits and seeds. The psyllium in some fiber products is a good start, but you certainly need more than just the one source. Other beneficial fiber supplement ingredients are flax and oats. You can even get soluble fiber from vegetable gums, such guar gum, acacia, and xanthan gum. These ingredients are often added to foods because the water they absorb improves the texture and feel of the food.

As you begin to make changes in your diet, you really shouldn't need to keep adding fiber as a supplement. Change your usual breakfast from a bowl of cereal and glass of orange juice to a bowl of oatmeal (real oatmeal, not the instant kind) with berries. Then make your afternoon snack a handful of nuts or popcorn, and you're already halfway to a healthy daily amount of fiber.

When you add fiber to your diet—either through foods or supplements—do so slowly. If you haven't been getting adequate fiber for a long time, your body probably isn't producing enough of the enzymes needed to break down the fiber, and this could result in excess gas. You can also try plain anise. It's a tonic that helps to settle the digestive system and expel gas. If you've ever eaten in an Indian restaurant, you've likely been served a small spoonful of anise seeds at the end of your meal. They're offered for more than just the flavor.

Please turn the page for your action plan for constipation.

⮞ Your Action Plan for Constipation ⮞

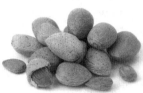

1. **To promote healthy digestion with no constipation, eat lots of fiber-rich plant foods**, including fruits and vegetables, beans, nuts, seeds, and grains. Aim for 30 grams of fiber per day.

2. **Drink at least 8–10 eight-ounce glasses of water daily.** This will promote proper digestion, help to bulk up your stools, and minimize gas and bloating as you increase the fiber in your diet.

3. **Exercise for at least 30 minutes, 5 to 6 times a week.** If you commit to a vigorous workout every day, you'll reduce your risk of constipation by about 40 percent.

4. **Take top-quality probiotics regularly**, to replenish the population of healthy bacteria in your gut. And eat lactic acid–fermented foods and live culture yogurts regularly to help them prosper. This step will not only help keep you regular, but also improve your overall digestive health and immune health.

5. **If you still find you are constipated, try a natural herbal laxative**, such as cascara sagrada, rhubarb, or triphala. But don't use a laxative for more than 2 weeks at a time. Take the lowest possible dose to reliably ensure a bowel movement each morning. Then, the next week, cut your dosage in half.

6. **Increase your fiber intake**, especially if you are taking a laxative. Try doing this mainly with fiber-rich foods, but you can add a fiber supplement, too, if necessary.

7. **Retrain your bowels** by attempting a bowel movement at the same time every day, preferably immediately after breakfast or exercise.

8. **Never repress an urge to defecate.**

9. **Talk to your doctor about the prescription and over-the-counter medications you take** on a regular basis to see if they are contributing to your problem.

❖ ❖ ❖

You now have the details on 5 of the most common and debilitating symptoms associated with digestive dysfunction— heartburn, indigestion, nausea, excessive gas, diarrhea, and constipation. Together with the tools and techniques you learned for building a solid digestive health foundation and addressing the most common digestive conditions plaguing our population, you have what you need to create your own life-long digestive wellness.

In the next, and final, chapter, I'll give you my recommendations for keeping up the good work you've started here so you can enjoy digestive freedom, now and forever.

•••••••••••••••••••••••Track Your Success!••••••••••••••••••••••

To track your success with this Action Plan, I highly recommend that you record the exact steps you're taking to address your constipation each day, as well as the symptoms you are experiencing at the time, and how you are feeling emotionally.

Putting these details on paper is an excellent way to see what works for you. It's also a great way to document the improvements you're experiencing and just how far you've come using safe, natural solutions to your digestive problem.

Turn to pages 135–136 for sample pages that makes tracking this information simple. Use these pages as your master copy and photocopy more pages to fill in with your details.

PART IV

Digestive Freedom, Now and Forever

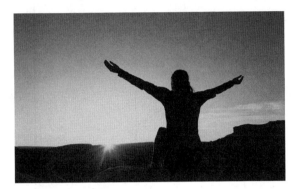

Congratulations! You've taken an important leap forward in finding safe, natural, proven solutions that can help you rebuild a strong, capable digestive system.

From having a better understanding of your amazing digestive system and all that it does for you, to learning about little-known tips, tools, and techniques for addressing your most pressing digestive concerns and the symptoms that go along with them, you now have the power and know-how to take action and secure your own digestive freedom. That means freedom from the physical discomfort and pain, as well as the emotional distress and worry that digestive ailments can bring.

As I've mentioned throughout this book, it's a good idea to track your efforts on paper so that you can remember exactly what steps you've taken toward your goal of better digestive health and resolution of specific digestive ailments.

It will also let you see—in black and white—the improvements you are feeling and just how far you've come on the road to digestive wellness. Sometimes the changes you experience will be dramatic, but other times they'll be subtle.

Writing everything down will give you a better awareness of and appreciation for each improvement. And it will increase your chances of having those "ah-ha!" moments, when you suddenly connect the dots from your past experiences and see clearly a new path for enhanced good health.

On the following pages are samples of my Tracking Sheet that you can use to record your efforts and progress. Use these pages as your master copies and photocopy more to fill in with your details.

Digestive Health Tracking Sheet				
Date	Condition	Action Step Taken	Symptoms I'm Feeling	Physical/Emotional Changes

Digestive Health Tracking Sheet				
Date	Condition	Action Step Taken	Symptoms I'm Feeling	Physical/Emotional Changes

PART IV

Give Yourself a Digestion Tune-Up Each Year

One last thing I'd like to recommend is that you consider an annual digestive system detoxification. It will help clear dangerous toxins from your body and rejuvenate critical organs and systems so that they can function more effectively and you can live with more vitality.

A regular detoxification will help you feel more comfortable, regular, energetic, focused and balanced. It will work hand in hand with all the other steps I've outlined for you in this book to improve your digestive function and overall wellness. And it will help you ensure that your digestive system is operating at top efficiency.

Detoxify gently

A gentle detoxification is good way to keep your digestive system on track and running optimally. On the other hand, harsh "cleanses" can damage delicate digestive system tissues, destroy the friendly bacteria there, and drive toxins that are traveling through your bowels deeper into your body. Clearly, choosing the right method of detoxification is essential. Following is what I suggest you do.

Start with an herbal laxative and natural fiber supplement

Begin your digestive system detoxification by stimulating your colon with an herbal laxative. This type of laxative is quite different from those I discussed earlier that are used for colon cleansing prior to a colonoscopy.

As I discussed in the Constipation section, an herbal laxative is gentle and tends to produce results within six to eight hours after you take it. For this reason, I suggest you take it at night just before going to bed so you'll be "ready to go" about the time you get up the next morning. Use the herbal laxative for two weeks. I recommend triphala, the popular Ayurvedic remedy that's a combination of three herbs—amla, beleric myrobalan, and *Terminalia chebula*. It's available in most health food stores and from numerous online retailers.

At the same time, supplement with a natural fiber product containing citrus pectin, oat bran, or psyllium. This is important for two reasons. First, the additional fiber gives your bowels something to push against while being stimulated with the herbal laxative. Also, when wetted, the fiber nutrients form a gel that helps to help pull old waste and contaminants out of the nooks and crannies in your colon. These toxins then bind with fiber in your stools, which allows them to be safely ushered out of your body.

Good natural fiber products to consider are Super Fiber Psyllium Seed Husk Powder from Country Life (*www.vitaminshoppe.com* or 1-800-293-3367).

Note: Be sure to increase your intake of pure, clean water when you're taking laxatives and fiber. Otherwise, the fibrous gel can become thick and cause an obstruction in your bowel rather than help with elimination.

When you use an herbal laxative and natural fiber supplement for two weeks, you'll notice a change in your elimination routine. Your bowel movements with likely be more frequent, larger, and easier to pass. Your urine output will likely increase as well, due to your increased water intake. Both of these changes will enhance the effectiveness of your digestive system detoxification.

Follow with restorative aloe vera extract

Once you've gone through the process of getting your intestines cleaned out, you need to restore your gastrointestinal tract, especially the gut wall itself, so it can do the job it needs to do in keeping toxins and digestive debris from being reabsorbed into your body.

One of the most healing substances for your skin is aloe and, as you've learned in this book, it's an important healer for the "inner skin" of your gut, too. The gel from the inner aloe leaf is high in antioxidants that target the digestive tract, and research suggests that aloe also improves bowel transit time and promotes a favorable balance of bacteria in the colon.

Use a quality aloe vera supplement for two weeks following your two-week herbal laxative and natural fiber regimen. I recommend Herbal Laxative, which contains both cascara sagrada and rhubarb, from Thorne Research (*www.thorne.com* or 1-800-228-1966).

Tend to your liver, too

Because detoxification is an active process that can generate free radicals, it's important to support your body's number one detoxification organ—your liver. Also, your colon works in concert with your liver, so it makes little sense to cleanse one without the other.

The most well-studied herb used to promote and protect your liver is Silybum marianum or milk thistle. Research has shown that silymarin—the active ingredient in milk thistle—can prevent damage to liver cells from everything from alcohol to carbon tetrachloride, and also has the unique ability to stimulate regeneration of damaged liver cells.

Extracts standardized to 70 to 80 percent silymarin are the most effective and I recommend a dose of 150–300 mg, three times daily. You can find a variety of silymarin products in most health food stores. Follow labeled instructions and take your silymarin supplement for a total of four weeks to wrap up your digestive system detoxification.

Resources

AHCC

AHCC is a medicinal mushroom extract and one of the most common complementary cancer therapies. A recommended brand is ImmPower, which can be purchased from Harmony Company (*theharmonyco.com* or 1-800-521-0543).

Aloe Vera Concentrate

Aloe vera concentrate is a well-known nutrient for soothing and nourishing the walls of your digestive tract. Look for Aloe Life, Aloe Master, Lily of the Desert, and Aloe Ace brands of aloe vera concentrates in health food stores.

Avemar/ AvéUltra

Avemar is a fermented wheat germ product that is helpful for protecting and promoting your body's health during any phase of cancer treatment. It is produced in Budapest, Hungary, by Biromedicina. In the United States, the product is being sold under the name AvéUltra instead of Avemar, but otherwise it's exactly the same. It's available through The Harmony Company (*theharmonyco.com* or 1-888-809-1241).

Butyric Acid Enemas

A company called Tyler Encapsulations makes a kit that contains everything you need to give yourself butyric acid enemas for two weeks to help stop chronic diarrhea and restore a balance in the colon. The kit is available from Key Pharmacy at 1-800-878-1322.

Chia

Quality chia sources are Ruth's Hemp Foods (*ruthshempfoods.com* or 1-877-359-4508) and Natural Remi-Teas (*naturalremi-teas.com* or 1-866-428-0575).

Chlorophyll

Two top chlorophyll products that you can use to make aloe vera more effective in treating the inflammation of IBD are Nature's Way Chlorofresh and Bernard Jensen Chlorophyll. Both are readily available in most health food stores.

Citricidal

This natural quaternary compound is synthesized from the seed and pulp of certified organic grapefruit and deionized water. It's terrific for preventing and treating traveler's diarrhea and is available from NutriBiotic. You can find it in health food stores or you can get it directly from NutriBiotic (*nutribiotic.com* or 1-800-225-4345).

ColoSure™ DNA Home Test Kit

This colonoscopy alternative analyzes the DNA in your stool to determine whether there's evidence of genetic mutations that occur in all cancer cells. When a cancer grows in the colon, it sheds cells into the stool. ColoSure tests your stool sample for 23 DNA markers associated with colorectal cancer and pre-cancerous polyps and costs about $399 per kit. For more information, go to *dnadirect.com*.

Diamond V XPC

This yeast culture product, originally produced for livestock, can be used safely, effectively and affordably to enhance your immune system. It's available from Wholesale Feeds in Marion, Iowa. They don't take Internet orders, but you can call them at 1-319-377-5528. (Remember that the product is sold for animal use, so don't ask them questions about use for humans.) You can also try your local feed store. If they don't have the product, ask if they can order it for you.

Digestive Enzymes

These are available in most health food stores or you can contact Progressive Laboratories (*progressivelabs.com* or 1-800-527-9512). They sell an excellent product called Digestin #987.

Electrolyte Rehydrating Drink

Try HEED sports drinks by Hammer Nutrition. They are formulated for endurance athletes and are made from complex carbohydrates, sweetened with stevia and xylitol, provide a full spectrum of all-chelated minerals, and come in a variety of flavors. They can be purchased at numerous running, cycling, multi-sport, and outdoor outfitter stores. Go online to *hammernutrition.com* to find a dealer near you, or you can order direct from this site.

EpiCor

The immune-enhancing fermented yeast culture product from Diamond V Mills is available from quite a few suppliers, including Vitamin Research Products at *vrp.com* or 1-800-877-2447; and Healthy Origins, at *healthyorigins.com* or 1-888-228-6650.

Euro-Cuisine Yogurt Maker

This top-recommended yogurt maker can be purchased from a variety of online retailers.

Fruit and Vegetable Spray

To help eliminate chemicals, dirt, and germs from your fruits and vegetables, use Healthy Harvest Fruit and Vegetable Rinse Spray before you eat them. It's available at numerous grocery stores, health food stores, and through a variety of online retailers.

Ginger Root

Ginger root is excellent for helping to minimize or prevent nausea. But products can vary widely in quality and potency, so it's important to use ginger supplements from a reputable provider. Try Ginger Root from Penn Herb Company, Ltd. (*pennherb.com* or 1-800-523-9971).

Home Fecal Occult Blood Test Kit

EZ Detect, a home fecal occult blood test kit, is affordable and most insurance programs, including Medicare, pay for some colorectal screening. You don't need a prescription for it and you can order directly from *ezdetect.com* or by calling 1-800-854-3002.

Hydrogen Peroxide

A good hydrogen peroxide product to help eliminate pathogens in your gut that may be contributing to IBS symptoms is Aerobic 07 from Aerobic Life (*aerobiclife.com* or 1-800-798-0707).

Lactic Acid Yeast Wafers

These help with diarrhea and can be purchased through your health care professional, or from Standard Process (*standardprocess.com* or 1-800-558-8740).

L'Equip Juicer

L'Equip juicers are efficient, effective, and make the job of juicing and clean-up a breeze. A full range of models is available through numerous online retailers and department stores.

Modified Citrus Pectin

PectaSol and PectaSol-C are quality modified citrus pectin products. They come in powder form, which can be mixed with water or juice. PectaSol-C is also available in capsules (6 capsules are equivalent to 5 grams of powder). Both products are designed to be taken on an empty stomach, at least one hour before or after food. You can order PectaSol or PectaSol-C directly from EcoNugenics at *econugenics.com* or 1-800-308-5518.

Peppermint Oil Capsules

European studies have found that enteric-coated peppermint oil capsules are very effective in treating IBS. They're available in the United States under the name Mentharil by PhytoPharmica (*phytostore.com* or 1-877-241-8822). The dosage generally recommended for IBS patients is 2–3 capsules a day taken between meals.

Probiotics

Good probiotic choices are Acidophilus Pearls by Enzymatic Therapy (*enzy.com* or 1-800-783-2286) and Probiotic Advantage or Probiotic Advantage Extra Strength (both from *drdavidwilliams.com* or 1-800-888-1415).

Psyllium Husks

An excellent source for psyllium husks is Freeda Vitamins (*freedavitamins.com* or 1-800-777-3737).

Sialex

This product is an alternative to slippery elm and is available from Ecological Formulas. It contains an extract of mucin, the main component of mucus, which re-establishes the protective mucus layer in the bowel and provides a lubricating action. The recommended dosage is 1 to 3 capsules with meals. It can be purchased online from *Netriceuticals.com* or call 1-888-852-4993 to order.

Slippery Elm

You can purchase slippery elm in bulk or in capsules in most health food stores or from companies such as Penn Herb (*PennHerb.com* or 1-800-523-9971), or from Kalyx.com (*Kalyx.com* or 1-315-245-3000).

Sugar Alternatives

XyloSweet (Xylitol)

Xlear (*xlear.com* or 1-877-599-5327)

Stevia

Body Ecology (*bodyecology.com* or 1-800-511-2660)
The Heritage Store (*caycecures.com* or 1-800-862-2923)

"Traveler's Friend" Antidiarrheal

This formula is available form NutriBiotic. You can find it in health food stores or you can get it directly from NutriBiotic (*nutribiotic.com* or 1-800-225-4345).

Waterwise 9000 Water Distiller

The water distiller I recommend and use myself is the Waterwise 9000. Visit *waterwise.com* or call 1-800-874-9028 to order.

Endnotes

1   Lowes R. Every Tenth American Was Prescribed a GI Medication in 2007, Says Federal Agency. *Medscape Medical News*, February 12, 2010.

2   Sanchez A et al. Role of sugars in human neutrophilic phagocytosis. *The American Journal of Clinical Nutrition*, November 26, 1973:1180-1184.

3   *Calif Med* 56;84(1):39–42.

4   Orme-Johnson D. *Pschosomatic Medicine.* 1987;49:493–507.

5   Fassa P. Learn All About Sleep and Its Connection with Your Immune System: *naturalnews.com*, July 17, 2009.

6   2009 *Sleep in America Poll*, National Sleep Foundation; March 2, 2009.

7   *Gut* 04;3(12):1730–1735.

8   *Gut* 04;53:1070–1074.
    Am J Gastroenterol 05;100:2616–2621.

9   SDI/Verispan, VONA, Full year 2008.

10 National Digestive Diseases Information Clearinghouse, National Institute of Diabetes and Digestive and Kidney Diseases, National Institutes of Health. *Smoking and Your Digestive System.* Publication No. 06-949, February 2006.

11 Oqbru O. and Marks J. Nonsteroidal Antiinflammatory Drugs (NSAIDs) and Ulcers. *MedicineNet.com*, January 30, 2007.

12 *J Infect Dis* 99;179(6):1523–1530.
    Am J Gastroenterol 00;95(9):2306–2311.

13 *Semin Thorac Cardiovascular Surg* 03;15(2):158–166.
    Nippon Rinsho 02;60(8):1639–1643.
    Gastroenterol Clin North Am 02;31(2):421–440.

14 *World J Gastroenterol* 05;11(33):5180–5184.
    J Physiol Paris 97;91(3-5):151–171.

15 *Dig Dis Sci* 95;40:576–579, 580–583.

16 *Vrachebnoe Delo* 88;2:79–81.

17 *J Gastroenterol* 01;36(2):91–95.
    Neuroreport 97;8(9-10):2305–2309.
    J Pineal Res 05;39(4):375–385.

18 *Gastroenterology* 02;123:2108–2131.

19 *Am J Gastroenterol* 03;98(6):1348–1353.

20 *Br Med J* 79;835–836.

21 *Turkish Journal of Gastroenterology*, March 2007.

22 Achkar J. *Inflammatory Bowel Disease,* The American College of Gastroenterology, *gi.org*, 2010.

[23] Ibid.

[24] Tresca A. *Colon Cancer and IBD Are You at Risk?*, About.com Guide, April 10, 2010.

[25] *American Journal of Gastroenterology*, online April 6, 2010.

[26] Kellog JH. *Colonic Hygiene: Comprising New and Important Facts Concerning the Physiology*, Good Health Books, 1915.

[27] Chan AO, et al. Prevalence of colorectal neoplasm among patients with newly diagnosed coronary artery disease. *JAMA* 07;26;298(12):1412–1419.

[28] Achkar J. *Inflammatory Bowel Disease*, The American College of Gastroenterology, *gi.org*, 2010

[29] National Cancer Institute, U.S. National Institutes of Health, Annual Report to the Nation Finds Continued Declines in Overall Cancer Rates: Special Feature Highlights Current and Projected Trends in Colorectal Cancer, *cancer.gov*, December 7, 2009.

[30] Ibid.

[31] *Pathol Immunopathol Res* 86;5:286–296.
Immunopharmacology 99;41:89–107.
Eur J Immunol 91;21:1755–1758.)

[32] *FASEB J* 06;20(4):A143.

[33] U.S. Centers for Disease Control and Prevention, news release, April 15, 2010.

[34] The Harvard Medical School Family Health Guide, *Preparing for a colonoscopy*, health.harvard.edu, 2006.

[35] *Br J Cancer* 03;89:465–469.

[36] *Hepatogastroenterology* 00;47:393–395.

[37] *Magy Seb* 04;57:168.

[38] *Pharmindex Handbook of Oncology* 2004/2005. CMP Budapest, 2004. p. 611–617
Cancer Biother Radiopharm 99;14(4):277–289.
Cancer Biother Radiopharm 04;19(3):343–349.
Cancer Biother Radiopharm 04;19(6):746–753.

[39] *Anticancer Res* 98;18:2353–2358.
Cancer Biother Radiopharm 99;14(4):277–289.

[40] *Altern Med Rev* 00;5:546–552.

[41] *Clin Med: Oncol* 07;1:73–80.

[42] *J Appl Physiol* 03;95:491–496.

[43] *Anti-Cancer Drugs* 98;9:343–350.
Biotherapy 01;12(3):303–309.
Int J Immunotherapy 95;11(1):23–28.

[44] UNICEF, The State of the World's Children 2008: Child Survival. p. 8. ISBN 978-92-806-4191-2, December 2007.

[45] Fujimoto GR, Robin MR, and Dessery BL. *The Traveler's Medical Guide*. Saint Paul, MN: Prairie Smoke Press. 2003.

[46] *Med Ann Dist Columbia* 61;30:326–328.